Ultimate Cancer Treatments

Alternative help for sufferers and their families

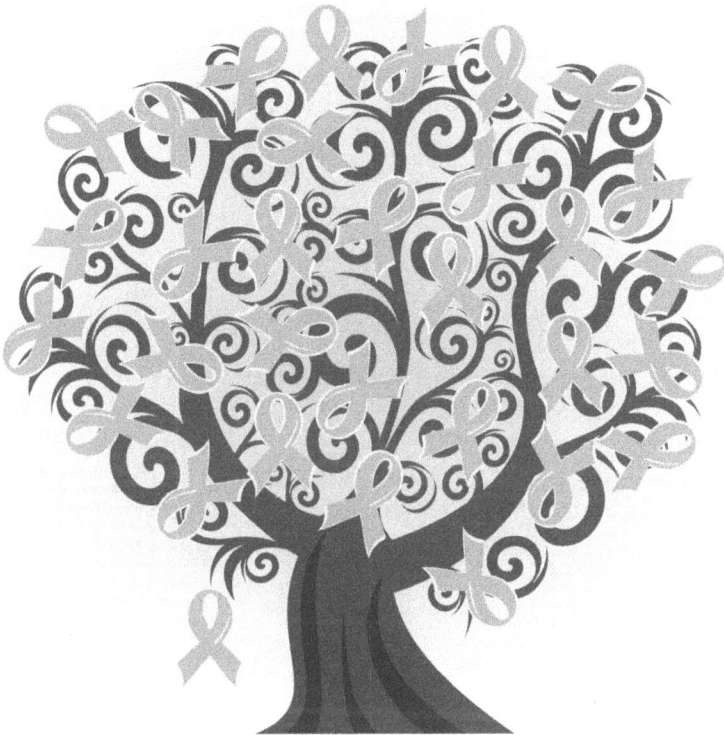

PATRICK JOYCE & HENRI SANT-CASSIA

"Myths busted, scam treatments exposed."
"The complete alternative cancer remedy guide."
"Maximize your survival strategies."

ISBN 978-0-578-09298-0
Library of Congress Cataloging-in-Publication Data: 2011939593
Patrick Joyce & Henri Sant-Cassia
Includes Bibliographical References
1. Cancer-Alternative Treatment. 2. Cancer-Treatment. 3). Cancer-Popular Works.

The authors of this book are not physicians. The information presented in this book is no way intended as medical advice or as a substitute for guidance by your physician. Consult your physician before adopting the medical suggestions in this book. Although the authors and publisher have made every effort to ensure the accuracy and completeness of the information within this book, we assume no responsibility, liability, directly or indirectly for the information, errors, inaccuracies or any inconsistencies herein. Any slights of people, places or organizations are unintentional.

First Edition Published in San Francisco, CA, USA by TouchStone Enterprises, LLC

This book is dedicated to Haley and Aidan,

who are my greatest teachers, and inspire me to be my very best

and to contribute great things to this world.

ABOUT THIS BOOK

This is a living book. We continually assess alternative cancer treatment developments, cutting-edge remedies and all the evidence to back-up the claims. We regularly consult with top cancer experts to stay on top of this field.

Most importantly, this is a long term commitment for us. We welcome feedback, stories and information from our readers and will incorporate all new knowledge into every subsequent edition.

This book comes with a money back guarantee. We are not in the business of making hard sales to anyone burdened with an illness. So, if you read this book and don't come out better informed at the end of it, we'll refund the cost of the book.

We believe in quality and guarantee that we have put together the very best book on alternative cancer treatments on the market. To learn more, go to www.Ultimate-CancerTreatments.com.

Email us with feedback, stories or questions: info@UltimateCancerTreatments.com.

Visit our website: www.UltimateCancerTreatments.com.

CONTENTS

INTRODUCTION

Nothing casts a deep shadow quite like cancer. Fatal outcomes, false information and a bewildering variety of possible treatments can create confusion, anxiety and fear at a time when you are looking for confidence and hope. For those facing this journey, perhaps the biggest kick in the gut is the moment when you discover that conventional Western medicine can go no further with your case. For those who reach this point, there are many myths, traps and outright scams which can mislead you, costing you valuable time, energy and funds. However, there is hope and some solid, viable ways to improve your chances for recovery.

The world is littered with products that make bold claims about curing cancer and offer no sound evidence. Moreover, outside tightly controlled pharmaceutical markets, there aren't any standards and controls. From natural remedies, to state-of-the-art formulations, there are a lot of choices and very little reliable information to help you determine what is effective.

Solid information is hard to come by and there is a clear need for a totally independent, responsibly written, professionally researched guide. With this as our goal, we studied the foremost treatments recommended and sold today. We studied the published clinical evidence, the theory behind the treatments and the known effects to date. Within these pages, we offer our findings as a quick and reliable resource.

We expose purported cures that have no discernable effect and that may actually be harmful. Our efforts are intended to quickly lead you to the best possible solutions and assist you with your decision making.

What we found were a handful of truly useful possibilities, as well as many scams and myths. Picking through the clinical trials and getting to the bottom of the claims wasn't easy and demonstrated to us the maze that most patients find themselves in. Choosing an alternative treatment and assessing its risks and benefits is just as vital, as doing so when considering Western chemotherapy, surgery or radiation.

We brought all this research together into a simple, easy-to-use guide. Each possibility is explained, and we give a clear verdict on how effective each might be.

Everything from the product and practitioner contact information, to the cost of the treatment is clearly identified. You can learn, compare and contrast your best options, and thus make aware and informed decisions.

Much of the information currently available to sufferers is generated by vested interests in the medical or pharmaceutical industries. It is also designed to market for sale and not to inform responsibly. We have checked most every study and statement carefully. We are totally independent from any commercial entity involved in selling treatments and our research base is peer reviewed and referenced.

We aim to make alternative cancer treatments a safe and effective option for sufferers. Learn the TRUTH about the most popular treatments which you are likely to consider.

PART ONE:

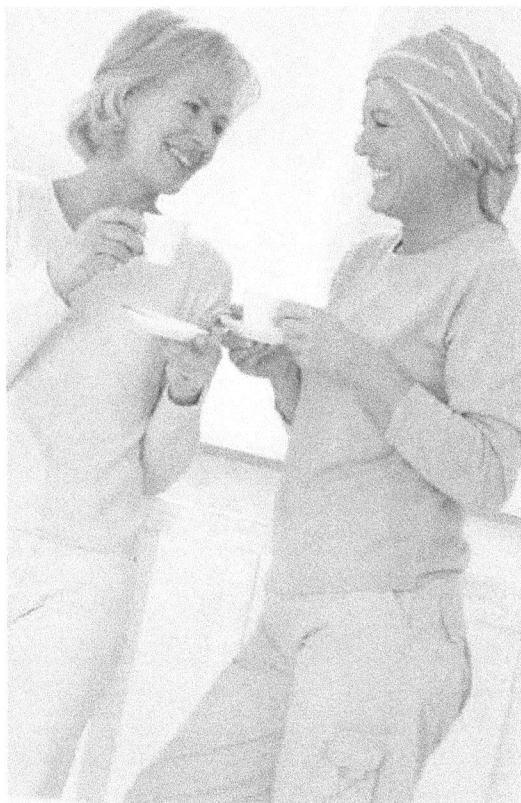

ALTERNATIVE CANCER TREATMENTS TO CONSIDER

T CELL GENETIC ENGINEERING

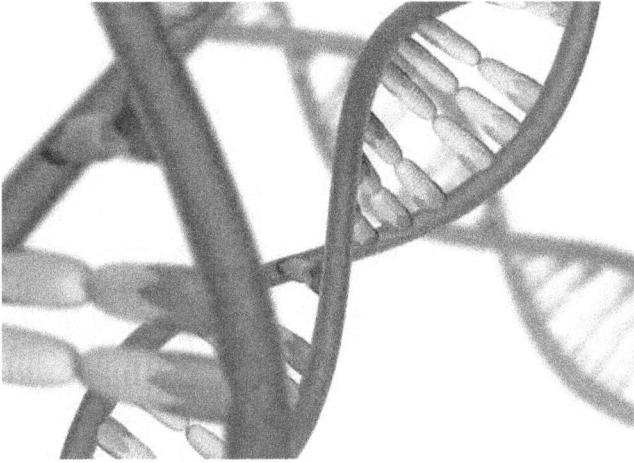

OVERVIEW

Genetically engineered T cells are at the forefront of exciting advancements in gene science and its application to cancer treatments. This method is an improvement on current practices in immunotherapy, which already uses injection or IV infusion of stem and immune cells to act as cancer vaccines in the body. It involves extracting the patient's naturally produced immune cells, injecting those cells with a genetically modified virus, and then infusing it back into the body. These reprogrammed T cells then transmit instructions to regular T cells to identify and attack all cancer cells. Furthermore, they duplicate themselves, becoming an army of killer T cells.

Although genetically engineered T cell treatment is currently undergoing clinical trials in the US, the results have electrified the research community. For example, the first three leukemia patients to undergo this treatment have experienced complete remission. These are spectacular results, as they were late stage patients who had shown resistance to conventional chemotherapy. The benefit for leukemia treatment is particularly tremendous, given that the current method of bone marrow transfusion is very risky and can be fatal for 20% of patients due to complications. However, the potential is not only limited to leukemia but to other forms of cancer cell lines as well. It should be noted, however, that this treatment is very new and relies on cutting edge gene science. Those interested in the treatment will most likely at this point only be able to obtain it through participating in a clinical trial.

MECHANISM OF ACTION

The mechanism of action revolves around genetically altering a virus that is able to carry instructions for T cells, consequently directing them to target leukemia cells. To do this, researchers used a unique molecule in leukemia cells that is absent in normal cells. This molecule serves as the target and was first identified by Dr. Lee M. Nadler, dean of Harvard Medical School. Using this target allowed them to program the virus to only attack leukemia cells—not normal cells—with the help of a chimeric antigen receptor (i.e., a protein that binds itself to the molecule identified by Dr. Nadler).

After the modification process of the virus was completed, it was injected into the T cell samples drawn from the patient with chronic lymphocytic leukemia. The T cells were infected by the virus, essentially becoming reprogrammed by the viruses' instructions. When reintroduced into the body, the T cells replicate and each of their chimeric antigen receptors bind with a cancer cell and kill it before moving on to the next cancer cell. According to research estimates, each T cell is able to kill thousands of cancer cells, and in total remove the equivalent of one kilogram of tumor tissue.

After remission, these genetically modified T cells remain in the body at high levels for six months—creating "memory" cells that can repopulate—should recurrence take place.

WARNINGS AND SIDE EFFECTS

Introducing genetically modified T cells in the body does not come without side effects. Listed below are the health risks and side effects seen with the treatment thus far:

1. Loss of B lymphocytes
B lymphocytes are another type of immune cell in the body. Unfortunately, they are also attacked by the modified T cells. Continued low levels of such lymphocytes can lead to increased vulnerability to various respiratory, gastrointestinal, and immune infections.

2. Tumor Lysis Syndrome
Tumor Lysis Syndrome is a condition caused by the breakdown of cellular waste products undergoing through apoptosis. When cancer cell death takes place at a rapid rate, patients may experience chills, nausea, and fever.

RESEARCH ON T CELL GENETIC ENGINEERING

The concept of using the body's own immune cells as a vaccine to fight cancer is not new and has been the prevailing philosophy in the field of immunotherapy.

There have been many innovative clinical studies in this particular field that have produced results. For example, treatment performed at the Fred Hutchinson Cancer Research Center in 2008, scientists removed specific anti-cancer T cells from a man with stage 4 melanoma. They then cloned them to the quantity of 5 billion cells and reintroduced them into the man's blood stream. The result was a complete remission.[1]

However, the method of generating tumor specific targeted T cells is limited because of the many varieties of cancer characteristics. The concept of T cell genetic engineering is thus particularly attractive, as it is potentially applicable across multiple cancer cell lines. In addition, this therapy was also seen as a needed innovation in leukemia, which is risky to treat and does not adapt well to most methods of cancer treatment. Early attempts to produce such virus-modified T Cells for use in leukemia failed, as the cells were not able to survive in the patient's body and duplicate themselves.

The University of Pennsylvania researchers were, however, able to improve by encoding improved instructions in their specially designed lentivirus to ensure the T cell survival and cancer-fighting action. The virus carried a chimeric antigen receptor, (i.e., a protein that specifically targeted a molecule in the leukemia cancer cell).

After an initial small dosage of the virus-modified T cells, they found that the T Cells were able to multiply more than 1,000 times and proceed to eradicate all tumor development, thus causing complete remission. The improved T Cells were also able to last at high levels for 6 months and continue to survive in the blood stream over a year from the treatment, thus preventing recurrence of the cancer.[2]

NECESSITY OF MEDICAL SUPERVISION

This form of treatment depends on advancements in gene science and immunotherapies, and will vary depending on the type of study and clinical trial. Those interested in this specific type of virus-modified T cell treatment should approach the University of Pennsylvania, while others more interested in immunotherapy on the whole can consult experienced immunotherapists to find out current methods for the various cancer cell lines.

Due to the lack of available scientific study regarding this realm of treatment, pregnant and nursing women will need to wait for further developments in this area of research. Early trials do indicate, however, that the condition of B lymphopenia may make this treatment unsuitable for expecting mothers needing to transmit immune functions to their children.

PRACTITIONERS

Abramson Cancer Center (Clinical Trials)
University of Pennsylvania
http://penncancer.org
3535 Market Street, Suite 750
Philadelphia, PA 19104-3309, USA
1-800-789-PENN

PRICE

Because of the innovation of this treatment, it is still undergoing clinical trials; therefore, no price has been established.

CHML

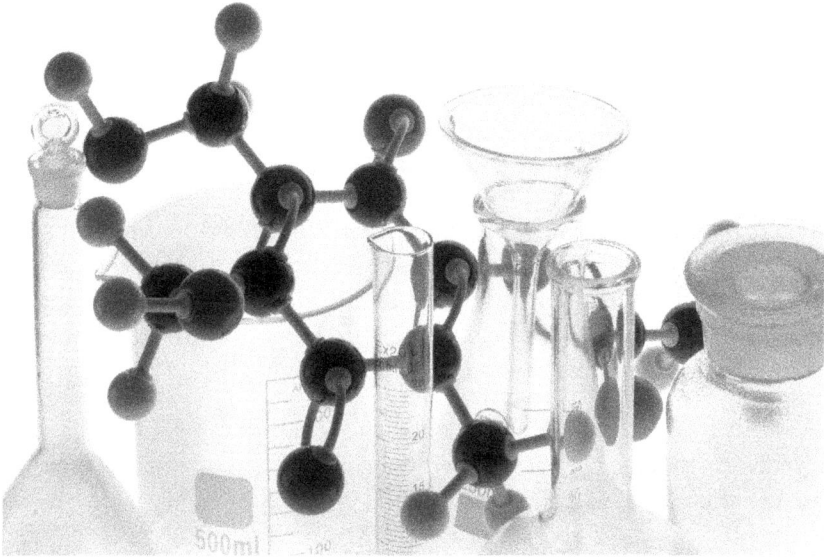

OVERVIEW

CHML, short for Cytotropic Heterogeneous Molecular Lipids, is a small-molecule anti-cancer drug developed by Chinese researchers that can penetrate the tough defenses of the cancer cells and induce apoptosis (programmed cell death), all without causing toxic side-effects. It is part of an emerging group of new biological treatments based on breakthroughs in the areas of nanotechnology and gene science. Although still undergoing review for use in the USA, CHML has already shown excellent results in Chinese clinical trials and been patented in many countries.

The problem with conventional anticancer drugs is that they are unable to get past the tough defenses put up by a cancerous tumor, which include a dense clustering of blood vessels, the strong collagen tissue in the interstitium, as well as the other components of tumor, before they can get to the cancer cells.

Advancements in nanotechnology, however, have made CHML 33,000 times tinier than a regular cell. Resistance is greatly reduced and CHML finds its way more easily into the tumor.

Its other great advantage as a treatment is that unlike traditional chemotherapy drugs, CHML is non-toxic and has no side effects. All components of the drug are isolated from organic ingredients and its composition mostly consists of fatty acids and lipid soluble vitamins.

MECHANISM OF ACTION

Apoptosis or programmed cell death plays an important biological function in our body by causing the death of defective or harmful cells in the body. Regular apoptosis functions tend not to be able to destroy malignant living cells like cancer, or to put a stop to degenerative diseases that kill healthy cells.

Researchers have discovered the individual sets of genes that program the process of cell death through certain encoded proteins or proteases. Namely, they are the caspase gene family and the BcL-2 gene family. The caspase set of genes are responsible for effecting the apoptosis pathway in dying cells while the BcL-2 genes control and stop this process from happening to living cells.

CHML works by directly manipulating the encoding processes of the caspase and BcL-2 gene sets to target diseases which poorly regulated by normal apoptosis. In the case of cancer, CHML can block the BcL-2 function in the living cancer cells and activate the caspase proteins to carry out the cell death pathways.

WARNINGS AND SIDE EFFECTS

CHML is non-toxic as it targets cancer cells only and does not destroy regular cells. Few effects have been reported in clinical trials of over 500 patients, the majority of these being low-grade nausea.

RESEARCH ON CHML

Research has shown the ability of CHML to suppress the growth of tumor cells at a non-toxic concentration of 25 to 100 mg/ml. When tested on strains of breast carcinoma, colorectal carcinoma, kidney carcinoma, lung carcinoma and myeloid leukemia, 6 hours of treatment at 50 mg/ml produced a 50% inhibition, while at 100 mg/ml; the effect was a 90% cell death rate. In contrast, non-cancerous skin fibroblasts were less inhibited in growth, supporting this hypothesis that CHML particularly suppresses tumor cells.

In terms of inducing apoptosis, CHML was able to trigger cell death in breast carcinoma, colorectal carcinoma, lung carcinoma and myeloid leukemia after 8 hours of treatment at 75 mg/ml. Results also seem to point towards apoptosis occurring through multiple pathways and not solely depending on the p53 protein.

Clinical trials conducted in Chinese hospitals between 1997 and 2003 treated 135 stage III and IV patients with liver and colorectal cancer, the majority of whom had received prior treatment and had ceased to respond to conventional treatment. 23% of liver cancer patients who completed the treatment experienced complete remission rate of 23%, while 54% saw partial remission. 20% showed no response and less than 5% showed progression. These rates were similar for colorectal cases.

NECESSITY OF MEDICAL SUPERVISION

CHML is a sophistical medical treatment method created using breakthroughs in gene science. It must be carried out by authorized medical practitioners in facilities that are equipped for the treatment. Administration can be conducted by IV drip, local injection or by a new method called Digital Subtraction Angiography (DSA) which delivers CHML directly to the tumor by Arterial Infusion. DSA can only be carried out by licensed radiologists.

CHML has the ability to inhibit cell growth as part of its process, which may not make it a suitable treatment for pregnant and breastfeeding women. There is also insufficient clinical data, which is why this group should not seek this treatment.

PRACTITIONERS

Glory Pharmaceuticals
http://glorypharma.com
2771 Manhattan Place
Vienna, VA 22180, USA
703-204-1703

PRICE

The treatment is not widely available yet as it is under review by the FDA for use in the USA. Contact Glory Pharmaceuticals for information on participating in a US-based clinical trial or a private treatment at an offshore clinic. The procedure is expected to cost about $25,000.

UKRAIN

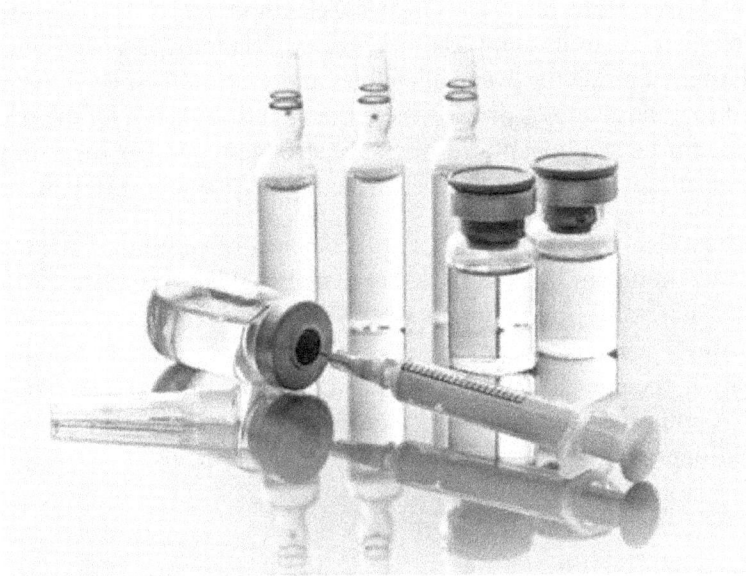

OVERVIEW

Ukrain is a synthesized anti-cancer drug created from the plant Greater Celandine (Chelidonium majus L). Ukrain is most commonly administered through injection or IV, and was praised by the late Dr. Robert Atkins as being a non-toxic alternative to chemotherapy.

Ukrain was discovered by a Ukrainian scientist Jaroslaw Nowicky while researching into the use of Greater Celandine as an Eastern European remedy.

Pre-clinical and clinical studies conducted in the 1990s have suggested that Ukrain is effective in fighting a wide range of over 60 types of cancers by completely inhibiting tumor growth and causing cancer cell apoptosis (programmed cell death), while having no toxic side effects. In addition, it seems to act as a biological response modifier (BRM) by boosting the body's immunity.

Ukrain's effectiveness, however, has been challenged by the scientific establishment and the creator of the drug has had difficulty licensing the drug internationally. While Ukrain is approved for use in UAE, Mexico and Eastern Europe, it has only been given orphan drug status in Australia and USA to be used on pancreatic cancer. People seeking to use Ukrain for other forms of cancer must consult with practitioners who provide the treatment.

MECHANISM OF ACTION

Ukrain is derived from the plant Greater Celandine, which is known to have a number of alkaloids in its composition. Greater Celandine has been traditionally used in Eastern Europe for liver, gallbladder and gastro digestive ailments, and it is believed that the alkaloids provide these therapeutic benefits. Of these alkaloids, chelidonine (or benzophenanthridine) is the strongest, and has the ability to stop spasms and stimulate the immune system, acting as a hepatoprotectant.

The actual mechanism of Ukrain is still the subject of continuing phytochemical research. The dominant hypothesis is that that alkaloids manipulate the metabolic activity of cancer cells by causing both regular and cancer cells to increase oxygen usage. However while oxygen usage quickly returns to normal in healthy cells, in cancer cells, it becomes severely inhibited. At the same time, Ukrain oxidizes their RNA, DNA and protein building blocks, preventing growth. The end result is that the oxygen-deprived and damaged tumor cells enter apoptosis.

WARNINGS AND SIDE EFFECTS

Clinical studies have shown Ukrain to be non-toxic, with side effects being a burning sensation, increase in temperature and more rarely, bleeding. There are no known reports of complications or fatalities occurring with intravenous use of Ukrain therapy.

However, strong warnings must be issued with the use of greater celandine, especially when self-administered orally. Due to the limited availability of Ukrain and its high costs, a number of people buy Greater Celandine extracts for consumption as a diet supplement.

Greater Celandine carries the following risks:

1. Hepatitis
Oral consumption of Greater Celandine has been associated with cases of acute hepatitis, not caused by any viruses or other substances, which ceased after the patient stopped taking the extract.

2. Allergies
Greater Celandine can trigger allergic reactions such as rashes, itching and potentially more serious reactions such as nausea and fever.

RESEARCH ON UKRAIN

A number of early pre-clinical and clinical studies largely conducted in Eastern Europe during the 1990s reported positive results on Ukrain as an anti-cancer drug treatment as compared to conventional treatments that included 5-fluorouracil and radiation, X-ray radiotherapy, Vitamin C, and gemcitabine. However, these studies have been challenged by Western authorities for being incomplete or lacking in a scientifically-recognized methodological approach. For example, the method of creating randomization was not sufficiently explained and researchers did not use recognized methods of statistics-testing. As a result, Ukrain was not deemed to have credibility as a drug by the mainstream scientific community.[3]

However, the drug's creator continued campaigning for the drug by making presentations at scientific conferences around the world, and has managed to spark continued interest in researching the drug in the last ten years, resulting in more credible studies published in peer-reviewed journals.

For example, two separate 2006 studies published in Anti-Cancer Drugs reviewed Ukrain positively and recommended it for further research. One tested Ukrain on Ewitng tumor cell lines and found that Ukrain inhibited cancerous cell growth, with a cytotoxicity comparable to the drug Etoposide. Another study[4] investigated the use on Ukrain on gliobastoma, a form of brain tumor, by testing three dosages on the genes and proteins involved with promoting the tumor growth of glioblastoma cells. Researchers found that there was a specific reduction in glioblastoma cell multiplication corresponding to the dosage. In addition, the expression of pro-cancerous proteins was down regulated. The study concluded that the drug may have therapeutic potential for brain tumors.[5]

NECESSITY OF MEDICAL SUPERVISION

As Ukrain is a medical drug that has to administered by injection or IV, those considering these treatments will need to seek out licensed medical professionals who provide the drug and treatment.

Due to insufficient clinical evidence on Ukrain and its effects on pregnancy and infants, pregnant women and breastfeeding women should avoid this form of treatment. They should also not take Greater Celandine in the light of potential health risk.

PRACTITIONERS

Jesse Stoff, M.D.
http://www.drstoff.com/
2-30 Beach 102nd Street #4B

Rockaway Park, NY 11694, USA
1-718-474-4734

Pangaea Clinic of Naturopathic Medicine
http://www.pannaturopathic.com
#120 - 12011 Second Ave
Richmond, BC V7E 3L6, Canada
1-604-275-0163

Reno Integrative Medical Center
http://www.renointegrativemedicalcenter.com
6110 Plumas St. Ste. B
Reno, Nevada 89519
1-775-829-1009
Toll-free: 1-800-994-1009

PRICE

As Ukrain is still little-known and not widely used, the costs are high. Ten 10-20mg injections of the drug will cost about $3,500, including the costs of shipment and medical care.

GRAVIOLA

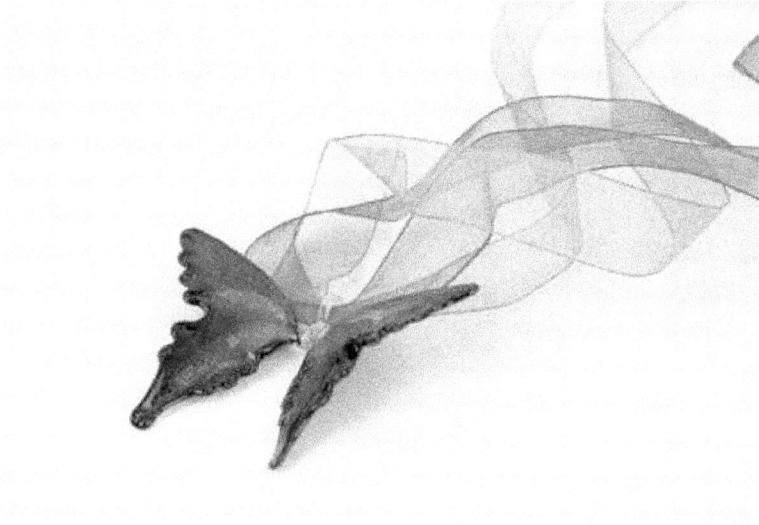

OVERVIEW

The graviola tree, found deep in the Amazon rainforest, has been known for centuries by the Amazon tribes as a healing tree, able to kill parasites and cure diseases. This drew the attention of researchers in the 1990s who discovered very powerful botanical compounds in graviola called acetogenins that are able to target and kill tumor cells in 12 different types of cancer without poisoning normal cells. If they can be developed into drugs, they would potentially be many times more powerful than current chemotherapy without the side effects.

The problem with graviola however, is that these powerful phytochemicals found in the living plant are difficult to synthesize into concentrated forms needed to fight cancer effectively. This is why Pawpaw, a related plant species with similar compounds, has overtaken it in terms of popularity amongst researchers.

However, although there has yet to been a breakthrough in harvesting graviola's full potential as an anti-cancer drug, the natural tree extracts are available and affordable since they cannot be patented, which make them a possible supplementary option in conjunction with a comprehensive cancer protocol.

The main manufacturers of graviola also produce another formula called N-Tense, which is 50% graviola and the other 50% a blend of seven other rainforest plant extracts with anti-cancer properties: mutamba, cat's claw, mullaca, guatonga, vas-sourinha and espinheira santa. Anecdotally, people who have used both prefer N-Tense to pure graviola as they feel the results are better with fewer side effects.

MECHANISM OF ACTION

Similar to Pawpaw, graviola is rich in annonaceous acetogenins, which are com-pounds that target cells in the body with very high energy consumption, typically malignant cells with DNA damage, cutting off their power and forcing them to enter apoptosis (programmed cell death). All this is done without harming any healthy cells.

Acetogenins are particularly effective with tumors that have built up strong defens-es to chemotherapy because they essentially plug the power supply to these cells, which receive energy through adenosine triphosphate (ATP) pumps. Without en-ergy, these tumor cells no longer have the power to multiply, build blood vessels or pump out toxic chemicals, making them more vulnerable to cancer-killing agents.

For this reason, acetogenins are considered to be part of the new wave of cancer treatments that will eventually become mainstream. Over 14 acetogenins that have this function have been identified so far by Purdue University researchers, of which a number are only found in graviola.

Continued research has also revealed that aside from its ability to cause apoptosis, graviola is able to regulate the overexpression of the epidermal growth factor recep-tor (EGFR), a gene that promotes breast cancer growth. By inhibiting this gene, the runaway processes of cell mutation that leads to cancer do not take place, and so cancer growth is either prevented or suppressed. Once again, this has no effect on other genes which regulate normal healthy cells.[6]

WARNINGS AND SIDE EFFECTS

Graviola has few reported side effects but there are a number of potential factors which should be considered when embarking on the treatment. There are also some supplements which counteract its effects and therefore should not be taken at the same time.

1. Nausea and vomiting
The most commonly reported side effect is nausea, which is common for large dos-es. Those who experience this can consider reducing the dosage or taking smaller dosages over the day with food.

2. Blood pressure problems

Although this has not been reported in human consumption, graviola has been shown to cause hypotension, vasodilation and cardiac-depressive symptoms in animals. So those with low and high blood pressure who are on medication should consult their doctors, and to check for any changes when taking the supplement.

3. Not to be taken with CoQ10, thyroid stimulators or antioxidants

Co-enzyme Q10 and certain thyroid medications work to increase ATP production which is not desirable as the objective is to starve cancer cells of energy, causing them to go into apoptosis. Antioxidants like Vitamin C and B varieties prevent apoptosis from taking place which is again, not desirable for this treatment, and will reverse the powerful effects of graviola.

4. Impact on gastrodigestive bacteria

Taking graviola over a long period of time may lead to the death of friendly bacteria in your intestines which help you with digestion. If you are contemplating long-term use, you should add probiotics and digestive enzymes to your diet so you can still enjoy the health benefits of these bacteria.

5. Risk of allergy

There is a rare occurrence of allergy to graviola, just as natural allergies occur with other forms of food.

RESEARCH ON GRAVIOLA

A 2002 study by Japanese researchers on one of graviola's main acetogenins, Annonacin, found that Annonacin performed better than the drug Adriamycin, which is commonly used in chemotherapy. As part of their study, lung carcinoma bearing mice were injected, Äîone group with Adriamycin and one group with Annonacin, with the third group acting as control.

Findings showed after two weeks that the mice injected with Adriamycin showed that tumors had shrunk by 54.6 per cent as compared to the control group, but 50% of the mice had also died from the treatment. In comparison, the group injected with Annonacin saw a reduction of 57.9 per cent, which is fairly similar to Adriamycin, but without any deaths or toxic effects.[7]

NECESSITY OF MEDICAL SUPERVISION

Medical supervision is not required for the self-administration of graviola supplements which are naturally derived and have no serious health risks. People wishing to take graviola should however be aware of possible side effects and only take it as a supplement with other cancer treatments.

Similar to Pawpaw, the acetogenins in graviola work by targeting cells with suspiciously high energy usage and starving them, which is why it is not suitable for pregnant or breast-feeding women.

PRACTITIONERS

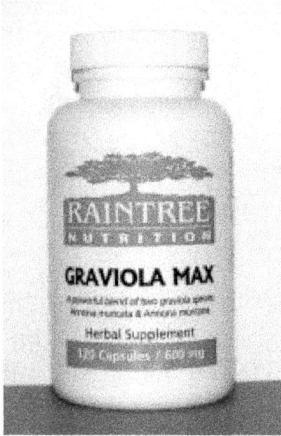

Raintree Nutrition
http://www.rain-tree.com
3579 Hwy 50 East, Suite 222
Carson City, Nevada 89701, USA
1-800-780-5902

Maximum International
http://www.maximuminternational.com
500 N.E. 25th St,
Pompano Beach, FL 33064, USA
Toll Free: +1-800-623-5333
Local: +1-954-623-5300

PRICE

The price of graviola extracts is about $20 for a bottle of 100 capsules. Variations include Graviola Max which incorporates Mountain graviola, and N-Tense, which combines graviola with seven other anti-cancer extracts. These products retail for about $30 for 160 capsules.

THE ISSELS TREATMENT

OVERVIEW

The Issels Treatment is an integrated Immunotherapy program that uses a combination of strategies to treat all types of cancers. Treatment methods include the use of surgery, vaccines, radiation, hormone treatment, a metabolic diet as well as a range of supplements.

The concept behind this approach is the belief that cancer is caused by unhealthy conditions in the body that lead to a dysfunctional immune, defense and repair system. Simply removing tumors and killing cancerous cells does not change the body's environment from promoting recurrence, which is why it seeks out a comprehensive approach to help "reset" the body's immune and regulating system to begin identifying and eliminating malignant cells again.

This treatment program was created in 1981 by Dr. Josef M. Issels, a German doctor who championed an integrative approach to treating cancer. Aside from his work in cancer treatment, Dr. Issels was a member of the German Federal Government Commission in the Fight Against Cancer up to his retirement in 1987. The Issels Treatment Centers are now run by his family, notably his son who is the chief specialist.

MECHANISM OF ACTION

The Issels treatment program mainly consists of two components: Specific and Non-Specific.

1. Specific Components
Specific components are the treatments that directly act towards removing and destroying cancer cells and tumors. These direct and targeted treatments include traditional methods such as surgery, radiation and chemotherapy, as well as unconventional methods such as hormone therapy and cancer vaccines.

Cancer vaccines
The vaccines are a unique feature of the Issels Treatment and essentially aim to work on invoking the body's immune response. Just as a chicken pox vaccine triggers a response by your body to build up its resistance to chicken pox, these vaccines stimulate natural cancer-killing cells such as interferon, monocytes, and others.

Examples of the vaccines used in the Issels Treatment include:

- Extracorporeal photopherisis with autologous dendritic cells (FDA-approved for T Cell Lymphoma)
- Coley's mixed bacterial vaccine
- Issels' autologous vaccine
- Lymphokine-activated killer cells and stem cells

It should be noted that while these promising vaccines have all been developed as the result of medical research and trials, that they do not guarantee success.

2. Non-Specific Components

Non-specific components form the more holistic treatment aspect that seek to recalibrate the body's environment, repair organ damage, and bring it back to a normal healthy state which can fight malignant cells on its own, and prevent recurrence. Typically these treatments involve a controlled metabolic diet and the ingestion of supplement. As the components are natural non-toxic substances, few side effects are noted.

Some features of these treatments may include:

- An organic immunity-boosting diet e.g. organic fruits and vegetables
- IV administration of nutrition supplements like anti-oxidants, minerals, vitamins and herbs
- Enzyme therapy
- Detoxification
- Psychological and emotional support groups
- Physiotherapy and exercise

WARNINGS AND SIDE EFFECTS

As the Issel treatment is customized according to the needs and medical history of the patient, there are generally no side-effects as dosages are adjusted to ensure that there are no adverse effects. In fact, it has been noted that the treatment usually alleviates the toxic side-effects of conventional cancer treatments like radiation.

It should be noted that the Issel treatment is very expensive, especially with some of their more exclusive treatments, so you should conduct more research before deciding to start this program.

RESEARCH ON THE ISSELS TREATMENT

Clinical research on immunotherapy notes that for the treatments to have maximum effect, the body must be restored to its regular, healthy state. Research suggests that vaccine therapy can have an impact not only on the immune system, but all the defense and regulatory mechanisms, especially in the connective tissues (pluripotent mesenchyme). However it should be noted that vaccine therapy has not been extensively researched for conclusive results on its effectiveness.

DENDRITIC CELLS

Dendritic cells are important regulating agents of the body's immunity, and they are responsible for adaptability of immune responses. One of their functions is identifying dangerous cells e.g. bacteria, cancerous cells and conveying those markers to T-lymphocytes which will then seek out those cells and destroy them. They are also able to distinguish between the body's own cells and the malignant ones, therefore informing the immune system which ones should not be attacked.

The Extracorporeal Photopheresis process channels blood through UV light, which separates immunity cells such as lymphocytes and monocytes from the blood. These cells are then cultured in a laboratory into active dendritic cells which are re-injected into the body as a vaccine.

AUTOLOGOUS VACCINE

The concept of the autologous vaccine is that each patient's blood is a reflection or representation of his or her unique body environment and cell culture. After studying the blood composition, the vaccine is prepared in the manner that will most promote the generation of immunogenic compounds within the body's internal environment.

NECESSITY OF MEDICAL SUPERVISION

The Issel treatment is only available at Issel treatment centers in the US and Mexico. Some of the treatments like the vaccines are not available outside of these authorized medical centers.

Due to the focus on immunotherapy, including treatment methods like vaccines and hormones, the Issel treatment is not suitable for pregnant and breastfeeding women.

PRACTITIONER

Issels Foundation Inc.
http://www.issels.com
8711 E. Pinnacle Peak Road, PMB 101
Scottsdale, Arizona, 85255
1-888-447-7357

PRICE

The Issels Treatment is very expensive as it includes inpatient residence at the treatment center. The total cost can range from $10,000 to $65,000.

VITAMIN B-17 (LAETRILE)

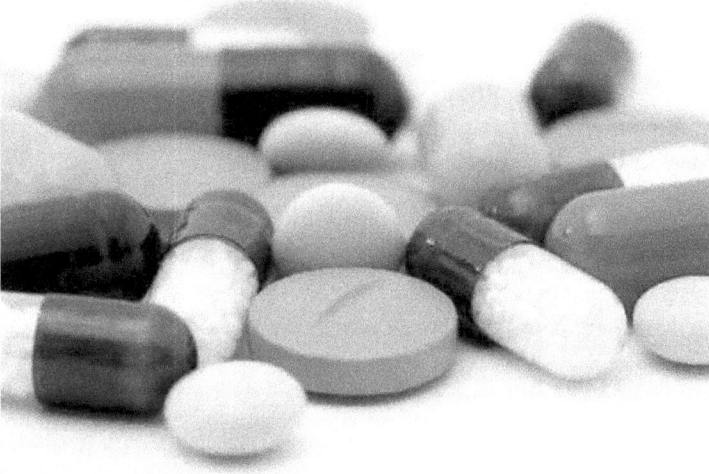

OVERVIEW

Vitamin B-17, or commonly known as Laetrile or Amygdalin, is a naturally occurring vitamin found in vegetables, most notably apricot kernels and other seeds. Originally isolated by French chemists in the 19th century, a purified version was produced by Ernst T Krebs, Jr., who named it Laetrile and started using it to treat cancer patients. It is one of the more well-known alternative cancer treatments, and is meant to be used in conjunction with a strict cancer-fighting diet and supplements like Vitamin B12 and C.

Laetrile performs a dual function of both destroying cancer cells and boosting the body's immunity in preventing future recurrences of cancer. However, it must be noted that Laetrile therapy takes a longer time to show effects, and should be combined with other cancer treatments as part of a metabolic therapy plan for best effects.

MECHANISM OF ACTION

The Laetrile compound, Laevo-mandelonitrile-beta-glucuronoside, breaks down into two separate glucose molecules: one of Hydrocyanide and one of Benzaldehyde. Either molecule has the effect of killing cancer cells, but both acting in unison produce a much more devastating effect.

Laetrile also encourages production of the enzymes Trypsin and Chymotrypsin in the body, which break down proteins protecting the cancer cell. When the cancer cell is exposed, they are more easily found and attacked by the body's white blood cells.

While Hydrocyanide and Benzaldehyde molecule is very effective against cancer cells, the difficulty with Laetrile is that the compound also chemically reacts with a number of enzymes in the body, for example Rhodanese, which breaks it down into a form that has no effect on cancer cells. To overcome this, Laetrile must be taken at high dosage and over a long period of time in order to interact with the majority of cancer cells.

Laetrile should be taken with supplements such as zinc, vitamin A, B (all forms), C, E, manganese, magnesium, and selenium. Pancreatic enzymes should also be taken to help laetrile molecules work at peak efficiency.

WARNINGS AND SIDE EFFECTS

The Food and Drug Administration strictly regulates the sale of Laetrile due to its views that Laetrile is not an effective treatment for cancer, although being a naturally found substance, it is not banned. While doctors are not banned from prescribing Laetrile supplements, they must make disclosure to the FDA. This has made Laetrile supplements unpopular with doctors in the US, although there are a number of successful practitioners in Mexico who use Laetrile treatment.

Laetrile supplements however are available on the Internet sold most commonly as pills or in liquid form for IV administration. It is also possible to consume the substance naturally by eating apricot kernels as part of a raw diet.

B-17 is water soluble and has no side effects. Reports of Cyanide poisoning have been reported to be a myth as Hydrocyanide molecules are digested and detoxified by the enzyme Rhodanese, and therefore do not build up in the body. The following warnings however should be noted by patients considering self-administration.

1. Possibility of Low Blood Pressure
The release of the Hydrocyanide molecule in the body is detoxified by the enzyme Rhodanese to become the thiocyanate molecule, which while non-toxic, can create a low blood pressure reaction in the body. This reaction is temporary, but should be noted by patients who have issues with their blood pressure.

2. Warning about Pancreatic Enzymes and Probiotics
As Pancreatic Enzymes are advised for patients on Laetrile, those embarking on this regiment should know that these enzymes are blood thinners, and should not

be used with other prescription blood thinners. Laetrile should also never be taken with probiotics as it may reduce the presence of Rhodanese to break down the Hydrocyanide toxin. In general, with any cancer-fighting regime, make sure that the supplements complement each other and will not cause any adverse effects.

ADMINISTRATION

Laetrile can be consumed in its natural form by eating the seeds of fruits like apples, apricots and peaches. In fact, this is recommended as a natural cancer prevention method. However, cancer suffers will require a purified version at a higher dosage, which is available as tablets and IV vials.

Cancer suffers are generally recommended to take 6 to 10 500mg tablets a day for the first month, before scaling down to 4 to 6 pills. While tablets can be self-administered, it is advisable for IV administration to be done by a nurse or doctor.

There have been no reported incidences of birth defects or abnormalities resulting from women who took Laetrile during pregnancy. However, caution should still be exercised given the lack of actual clinical trials.

RESEARCH ON LAETRILE

Studies on Amygdalin carried out in the 1970s on mice carrying mammary tumors found that the compound "significantly inhibits the appearance of lung metastasis" and the growth of the tumors. The effect of preventing new tumors was weaker; however the mice exhibited improvement in appearance and energy. Other studies supported the palliative effect of the compound, with current practitioners suggesting improved pain-relief and well-being in 60% of the cases.

It was also previously theorized that the hydrogen cyanide was the chief cancer-killing molecule that produced Laetrile's results, but research by Japanese scientists from Toyoma University (1980) has since shown that it is the benzaldehyde is the more effective cancer-fighting molecule.

NECESSITY OF MEDICAL SUPERVISION

No medical supervision is required for the consumption of Laetrile. Patients should do necessary research into the accompanying diet and supplements for best results. IV injections should be administered by a medical professional.

RETAIL SUPPLIERS

Apricot Power
http://www.apricotpower.com
720 South Main Street
Lakeport, CA 95453
Toll Free: 1-866-468-7487

Medicina Alternativa
http://www.tjsupply.com
416 W San Ysidro Blvd Ste L447
San Ysidro, CA 92173
Toll-free: 1-888-281-6663
Local: 1-619-819-7531

Our Father's Farm (Apricot Kernels only)
http://www.ourfathersfarm.com/
1050 Highway 5 West
Dundas, ON L9H 5E2
Canada
Toll-free: 1-888-946-8217
Local: 1-905-628-8195

PRICE

Ranging from $25 for a bottle of 100mg capsules to $85 for a bottle of 500 mg capsules. Also available in IV vial form.

HAELAN-951

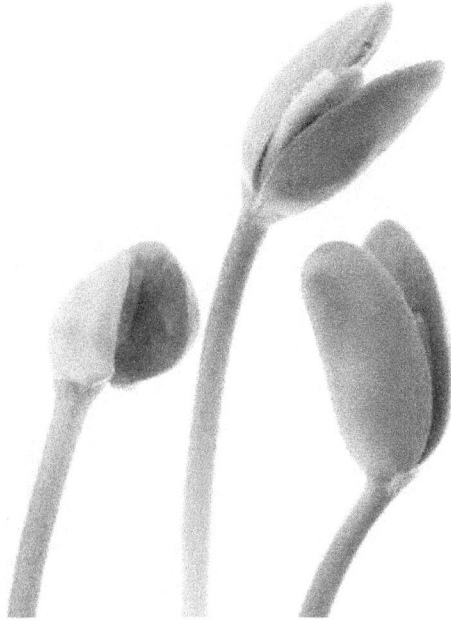

OVERVIEW

Haelan-951 is a fermented phytochemical soy supplement manufactured in China that has been receiving increasing recognition from doctors and consumers. Phytochemicals is an emerging field of research into the unique healing properties of plants that fight diseases and speed recovery, and soy is one of the most researched plants for its nutritional value. Although soy has long been known as a highly nutritious food with high levels of enzymes, amino acids and proteins, it has only been in recent years that researchers have discovered other important plant compounds like isoflavones, protease inhibitors, inositol hexaphosphate, saponins, and phytosterols that are not found in many foods.

Haelan-951 was created by a nutritionist working in a Chinese hospital as a means of liquid nutrition, and it was only when patients started to claim astonishing recoveries after drinking it that the drink came to the attention of cancer researchers. They found that the manner of its fermentation process had preserved very high levels of these active phytochemicals, including high numbers of protease inhibitors and isoflavones, which fight cancer. This process has since been patented and further refined to increase its nutritional value.

Haelan-951 has been recognized as an effective adjunctive supplement when used with other cancer treatments. As it has no active-cancer killing agents, it is not suitable for use on its own.

MECHANISM OF ACTION

Haelan-951 has a high concentration of protease inhibitors, which are hardy molecules that in plants, work to protect the species from disease and damage. In humans, they act to counteract proteases in the body that stimulate tumor growth in mutated cells. These protease inhibitors have a similar effect to chemotherapy in that they suppress cancer progression, but do so in a safe and non-toxic manner.

In addition, protease inhibitors act as antioxidants by neutralizing destructive free radicals in the body which cause stress and DNA damage. They help in DNA recovery, preventing damaged cells from mutating into cancer cells. These healing properties are most likely the reason for the restorative effects experienced by people who drink the supplement.

In addition, the other phytochemical agents also have anti-cancer properties: phytates which reduce the creation of free radicals, phytosterols which counter cholesterol waste, saponins which prevent cell mutation, phenolic acids which protect DNA from carcinogens, omega-3-fatty-acids which protect against disease, and lastly, isoflavones which can prevent hormone-related cancers such as breast cancer, ovarian cancer and prostate cancers. This is a new field of research and scientists are still trying to find out more about how these organic compounds behave in humans.

WARNINGS AND SIDE EFFECTS

Haelan-951 is certainly a therapeutic dietary supplement that should be considered as part of a cancer protocol but it should be noted that it is not an anticancer drug or a cancer cure, despite anecdotal claims of remission. There are also certain candidates for whom this supplement is not appropriate.

Estrogen-dependent breast cancer
Those with estrogen-dependent breast cancer are not advised to take Haelan-951 as there is debate over whether one of Haelan's isoflavones, Genistein, may counteract the drug Tamoxifen used in fighting estrogen-dependent breast cancer.

Soy allergies
Haelan-951 is also not suitable for those with soy allergies.

Other than the above, Haelan-951 has no side effects and has been shown to alleviate the toxic side effects of chemotherapy. Users should note that the product has a strong smell and is generally unpalatable.

RESEARCH ON HAELAN-951

A number of studies have been carried out on Haelan-951 and other soy products in the last 16 years. While initial research focused on the role of protease inhibitors and plant enzymes, more recent clinical research increasingly point towards the significance of isoflavones such as genistein and daidzein in Haelan-951's cancer-fighting properties. Aside from this, scientist have also discovered fatty acids called small biosynthetic anticancer agents in the supplement which also have anti-tumor properties, particularly the 13-methyltetradecanoic acid and 12-methyltetradecanoic acid which may contribute to apoptosis without killing normal cells.

It has been noted that in the clinical studies carried out by the manufacturer that notwithstanding low remission rates, all patients experienced improved well-being, appetite, sense of health and reduced nausea and other toxic side effects of chemotherapy and radiation treatments. This suggests that this product is best used along with chemotherapy as an adjuvant supplement, to help reduce the toxicity of the harsh cancer-killing treatments.

NECESSITY OF MEDICAL SUPERVISION

Haelan-951 is a natural dietary supplement that requires no medical supervision. As Haelan-951 is a natural fermented supplement that is free of side effects, it is safe for pregnant and breastfeeding women and may in fact be beneficial in replenishing nutrients in their body.

RETAILERS

Haelan Products, Inc. (Manufacturer)
http://www.haelan951.com
18568 142nd Avenue N.E., Building F
Woodinville, Washington 98072, USA
Toll-free: 1-800-542-3526
Local: 1- 425-482-2645

Gift of Haelan
http://www.giftofhaelan.com

Ultimate Cancer Treatments

7239 Turquoise Drive SW,
Lakewood, WA 98498, USA
253-582-5863

PRICE

Haelan-951 is available from the manufacturer at $60 per 8oz bottle (1 day's supply) and about $3000 for a two month supply. Importers and wholesalers may offer a lower cost for bulk orders.

MEDICAL OZONE

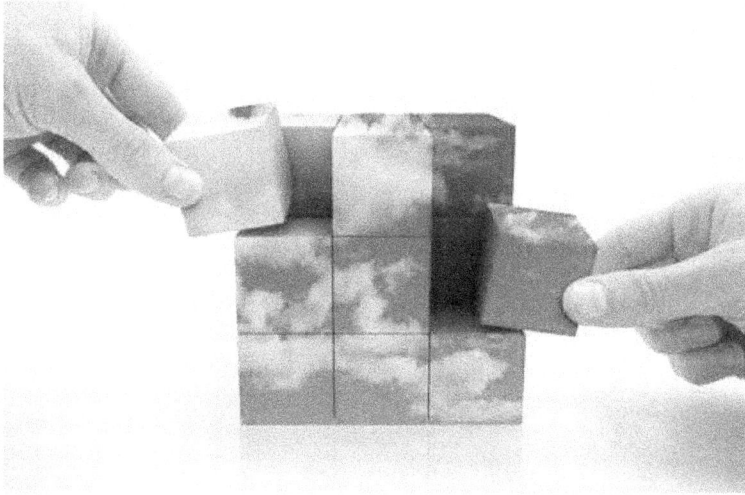

OVERVIEW

Ozone therapy is an alternative medical cancer therapy which involves infusing the body with ozone gas to flood the cells with oxygen, usually over a sustained period of time. The theory behind oxygen therapies comes from Nobel-winning scientist Dr. Otto Warburg, who found that when oxygen levels fall in cells, toxins build up, causing cells to turn cancerous. He advocated that to prevent cancer growth, cells must be able to respire and receive enough oxygen. Following from this, a number of treatment methods arose to raise the levels of oxygen in the body—of which, medical ozone is one of the most well-known.

Ozone is a toxic gas when inhaled, but when infused into the body, it has two major effects. Firstly, it has a strong oxidizing effect in the body, and is able to inhibit viruses, bacteria, and malignant tumors by oxidizing the toxins and dissolving their protective defense. Secondly, it provides oxygen to the cells, which may have been choked by the build-up of toxins and plaque in blood vessels and tissue. Ozone is also able to stimulate the body to produce more cancer-fighting immune cells like interferon and interleukin.

Research does indicate that ozone has beneficial effects. Medical ozone, however, is a controversial treatment due to disagreement over its validity and suitability as a treatment, as well as over the health risks. While ozone therapy is well-established in Europe and other countries, particularly Germany, Switzerland, Italy and Russia, as a complementary treatment, it does not have mainstream support and it is warned against by the FDA and the American Cancer Society.

MECHANISM OF ACTION

There is a variety of ozone treatments, which can be confusing. Essentially, the idea of ozone treatment is to maintain oxygen in the cells at a high rate consistently, so effectiveness relates to the frequency of the treatment, the concentration, and the way it is delivered. Those considering ozone therapy must also take note that oxygen levels should be slowly built up and not all at once to avoid shock.

While low levels of ozone are therapeutic, medical ozone is found to be most effective around the range of 27mcg/ml. Ozone treatment can be used for any part of the body except for the lungs and areas surrounding the lungs as the lungs are very sensitive.

Physician administered ozone treatments include the following:

- Direct IV injection of ozone: Ozone is slowly injected into the body once or twice a day at the rate of 1cc per minute up to the point where the body reaches saturation. Patients have to lie down throughout the treatment without moving so that the oxygen is allowed to disseminate.

- Autohemotherapy: This method involves circulating blood out of the body, infusing ozone through a machine and pumping it back to the body. This method is very safe, which is why it is the most widely used method in Europe.

- Extracorporeal Re-circulatory autohemo perfusion: This is an improvement on the autohemotherapy where blood is circulated out of the body, infused with ozone and filtered before it is pumped back into the body. This is a fairly safe method of delivering ozone as it prevents any inhalant. The filtering also traps oxidized waste products, helping to clean the blood flow in the process.

- In addition, the following self-administration methods are also used, although home-administration requires great care so as not to breathe in the ozone:

- Ozone-charged water: People can dispense small quantities of ozone into water and drink the water immediately. They must do this all day long whenever they drink.

- Ozone-bagging: People can purchase an ozone sauna suit and wear it to immerse the body in ozone gas from the neck down. Ozone is absorbed through the skin.

- Ozone steam cabinet: Similar to the ozone suit, the steam cabinet sprays or steams the body with humidified ozone for about 20 minutes.

WARNINGS AND SIDE EFFECTS

Despite ozone therapy being established in Europe as an alternative cancer treatment, in North America, it is not approved by the Food and Drug Administration, which considers ozone a toxic gas without any therapeutic benefits.

While the therapy itself is not illegal in the US, practitioners of ozone therapy operate under other many restrictions. For example, they can lose their medical licenses if they are seen to be marketing or promoting any forms of ozone therapy. In a much publicized controversy, Dr. Robert Atkins (who invented the Atkins Diet) announced on his New York radio show that he had cured a case of breast cancer by injecting ozone into the tumor. This prompted the New York State Medical Board to revoke his license, but the license was restored after public protest, on condition that Atkins ceased his promotion of ozone therapy. Ozone therapy is generally safe and non-toxic but the following health risks and side effects apply.

1. Risk of inhaling ozone
There is always the risk of ozone leakage during an ozone therapy session, particularly when the therapy is self-administered. Those considering ozone therapy should always take great care when using equipment.

2. Risk of gas embolism
Gas embolism is when air gets trapped in the blood as a bubble and can cause serious or fatal complications if it gets stuck in a blood vessel and blocks blood flow. Although incidence of this is low, there has been one known case of fatality in the USA due to air embolism after autohemotherapy.

3. Swollen veins, circulatory depression, fainting
Swollen veins is a side effect of having the machine pump blood out and back into the body, which can cause stress on blood vessels and can create circulatory depression. This is a temporary side effect.

4. Chest pain, cardiac arrhythmia and shortness of breath
The process can also cause a side effect of chest pain and arrhythmia, but this is less common.

RESEARCH ON OZONE

One of the few US-based studies found that ozone therapy was able to inhibit the duplication of breast, uterine and lung tumor after the cells were exposed to ozone for eight days. Ozone was able to inhibit cancer cell growth while healthy control cells were unaffected. Scientists concluded that cancer cells were less resistant to the oxidation capacity of ozone as compared to regular cells.[8] In terms of testing for toxicity, research in Italy on rabbits and healthy volunteers also showed that autohemotherapy stimulated increased production of immune markers while being non-toxic.[9]

More recently, 2004 clinical trial in Spain showed that ozone therapy was able to increase oxygenation in oxygen-deprived tumors, proving that ozone therapy was a more effective oxygen therapy than other known methods like hydrogen peroxide. In the study, eighteen patients were given ozone therapy via autohemotherapy thrice times in a week and oxygen levels in the tumor were tested using probes pre-therapy and post-therapy. Researchers found that the ozone therapy made the most difference with hypoxic (oxygen-deprived) tumors and low hemoglobin concentrations.[10]

NECESSITY OF MEDICAL SUPERVISION

There is ozone treatment equipment that allows people to self-administer the treatment themselves, but concentrated treatment methods can only be carried out by licensed and trained medical professionals. In any case, people considering ozone treatment should first consult their doctors as well as experts in this form of treatment for trained opinions.

While ozone therapy has been used on pregnant women, and practitioners feel that it is particularly useful in treating complications in pregnancy, the health risks and side effects remain a factor to consider. Those considering the therapy should consult with their physician and an experienced ozone therapist.

PRACTICIONERS

The Nevada Center of Alternative
and Anti-Aging Medicine
http://www.antiagingmedicine.com
1231 Country Club Drive
Carson City, NV 89703, USA
1-775-884-3990

Arrowhead Health Works
http://www.arrowheadhealthworks.com
27248 Hwy 189, Suite 8
Blue Jay, CA 92317, USA
1-909-338-3533

Oasis of Hope Hospital (Contreras Clinic)
http://www.oasisofhope.com
Paseo Playas No.19
Playas de Tijuana
Tijuana, B.C. Mexico
1-888-500-HOPE
1-619-690-8400

PRICE

Prices vary depending on the type of treatment, but typically range from $100 to $250 per session.

HYPERTHERMIA (ONCOTHERMIA)

OVERVIEW

Hyperthermia (also called oncothermia or thermotherapy) is a new type of cancer treatment that utilizes high temperatures (i.e., 107 °F - 113 °F) and radio frequency to kill cancer cells. Currently undergoing clinical trials, the treatment is seeing very positive results in terms of tumor reduction and remission when paired with conventional methods like radiation and chemotherapy.

While the benefits of heat treatment have been known for thousands of years, it was not successfully proven on a medical basis until the 1980s, when medical scientist James I. Birche proved that cancer cells broke down at high temperatures, while normal cells did not.

Hyperthermia is best used as an enhancer and is always paired together with conventional treatment methods, such as radiation and chemotherapy, usually within an hour of each treatment. After undergoing Hyperthermia, cancer cells that were not destroyed are much more sensitive to the effects of radiation and chemotherapy. This makes for a good way to target resistant cancer cells. In addition, Hyperthermia can also be used together with anti-cancer drugs to enhance their effects.

Although the treatment has gained legitimacy and popularity as a beneficial treatment, the science behind it is still not fully understood, which is why it is still the subject of current medical research. In recent years, technological breakthroughs in bio-engineering have evolved Hyperthermia as a reputable cancer treatment, as more advanced sensors, applicators, and magnetic nanoparticles are invented to heat the tumors more effectively.

Hyperthermia is most successful when used on localized cancers that are relatively close to the body's surface. Other methods offer less successful results.

CONTROVERSY

An early practitioner offering Microwave Hyperthermia was Dr. Kurt Donsbach, who developed the Al-Do Method with his partners, Dr. Rudolph Alseben and Cheung Laboratories. Dr. Donsbach claimed that aside from heating tumor tissue, his Pulse Modulated Microwave Hyperthermia could transmit encoded instructions that aid in tumor reduction. However, the clinic received complaints about its operating standards, and the clinic was shut down by Mexican authorities after the death of high profile cancer patient Coretta Scott King. Advocates of the clinic, however, noted that Coretta Scott King was already terminally ill and partially paralyzed when she arrived at the clinic after months of failed conventional treatments.

MECHANISM OF ACTION

One theory behind Hyperthermia's effects is that heating tissue causes cells to increase their activity levels. Increased cell activity calls for increased nutrition and detoxification, which normal cells can manage but cancer cells cannot, as they are already high energy users. If cancer cells cannot keep up, they may starve and undergo apoptosis.

Another theory has to do with blood circulation. When regular tissue is heated, blood flow can increase by up to ten times but the blood flow in tumors only increases by a few times. Also, when treatment is stopped, normal circulation is rapidly restored in regular tissue but the circulation in tumors becomes very slow. Multiple sessions of Hyperthermia may shock or overtax cancer cells and cause them to break down.

The effectiveness of Hyperthermia depends on whether temperatures are raised sufficiently to the level where cancer cells are destroyed, as well as other factors like the type of tumor and the duration of treatment. Currently, there are four types of hyperthermia treatment that being studied ‚Äì of which, localized hyperthermia is most effective.

Localized Hyperthermia

Localized hyperthermia involves applying heat directly to the tumor tissue. Firstly, local anesthesia is applied to the treatment area. Next, small needles or very thin thermometers are placed into the cancerous tissue to measure the temperature while the tissue is heated by microwave, ultrasound, or radio frequency.

Intra-cavity Hyperthermia

Although the localized method is easiest for a tumor that is close to the skin surface, there are methods to treat tumors that are located elsewhere in the body. For tumors inside body cavities like the throat and the rectum, probes can be inserted to heat the tumor. For tumors deeper within the body, the patient will need to be placed under general anesthesia while probes are inserted deeply into the body. Computerized imagining is necessary for this method so that the doctor can ensure correct placement. The heat source is then transmitted through the probe to deliver the heat.

Perfusion

Perfusion is a new technique being tried out in the treatment of larger areas of tissues like limbs or in larger organs. Under anesthesia, blood is drained out of the tumor, heated up and then circulated back into the organ. Anti-cancer drugs are often added in the process. For the abdominal cavity, another variation involves heating up anti-cancer drugs and pumping them into this cavity so that its temperature rises above 106 °F.

Whole-body Hyperthermia

This method is used only when cancer has spread throughout the body. Methods like thermal chambers or hot blankets are used to heat the entire body temperature. With the permission of a physician, patients may also carry this out in home saunas that are capable of reaching the appropriate temperatures.

WARNINGS AND SIDE EFFECTS

Temperature regulation

The temperature reached during hyperthermia is the most important factor in ensuring a safe procedure. As long as the temperature remains below 111 °F, most regular tissue will not suffer any damage.

This risk increases, however, when larger areas are being treated because of the larger range of tissues and cell structures involved. While the main area being treated may hit the right temperature, other areas may overheat and cause pain, blisters, or burns.

Side Effects of Perfusion

Due to the process of circulating heated blood and drugs, patients may suffer from some trauma to regular tissue like bleeding, swelling, or clotting. However, these side effects generally subside quickly after the treatment.

Side Effects of Whole-body Hyperthermia

The risks involved with whole-body hyperthermia are the highest. Exposing the body to high heat can cause side effects such as nausea, vomiting, and diarrhea, with some risk of cardio and blood circulation issues, although serious side effects are rare.

RESEARCH ON HYPERTHERMIA

Recent technological innovation has improved planning systems and modeling programs, which correspondingly allow for better design in applicators and monitoring systems. Also, medical breakthroughs have led to the creation of new application methods such as using gene therapy or vaccines together with hyperthermia, either to enhance anti-cancer effects, or to turn such mechanisms on or off.[11]

A recent example of a new technique is the use of magnetic nanoparticles and an alternating magnetic field to deliver the temperature. These nanoparticles are injected locally into the tumor and then controlled using a feedback temperature control system, which achieves accurate temperatures.[12]

A 2001 clinical trial found that whole-body hyperthermia was able to enhance the effects of Carboplatin (Platinum) in reducing tumors in patients who had platinum-resistant ovarian cancer. 14 eligible patients were treated every four weeks for six cycles, each time for an hour at 107 °F before the Carboplatin was administered. After the treatment, one patient saw a complete remission while four saw partial remission. Of the other nine, four had stabilized conditions; three saw their cancer progress while another two did not complete the treatment. This response rate shows that hyperthermia can overcome platinum resistance, which is promising news for this group of patients who cannot respond to treatment on its own.[13]

NECESSITY OF MEDICAL SUPERVISION

Hyperthermia is a medical treatment that requires special equipment and facilities. Therefore, people considering this method should seek out licensed practitioners, or apply to clinical trials being conducted.

Pregnant and breastfeeding women will not be suitable for hyperthermia treatments given the possible health risks and the necessity of radiation or chemotherapy.

PRACTITIONERS

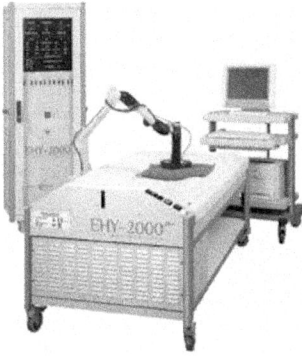

Arrowhead Healthworks
http://www.arrowheadhealthworks.com
27248 Hwy 189, Suite 8,
Blue Jay, CA 92317, USA
1-909-338-3533

Cleveland Clinic
http://my.clevelandclinic.org
2010 East 90th Street
Cleveland, OH 44195, USA
1-216-444-5571

Integrated Health Clinic (Canada)
http://www.integratedhealthclinic.com
2nd Floor - 23242 Mavis Avenue
Fort Langley, BC, V1M 2R4
1- 604-888-8325

PRICE

Hyperthermia is legal in the United States and Canada but not widely available, as it is still undergoing clinical trials. Patients opting for the treatments must accompany them with radiation. Costs vary but are believed to be about $16,000. Alternatively, patients can apply to on-going clinical trials.

INTRAVENOUS VITAMIN C (IV)

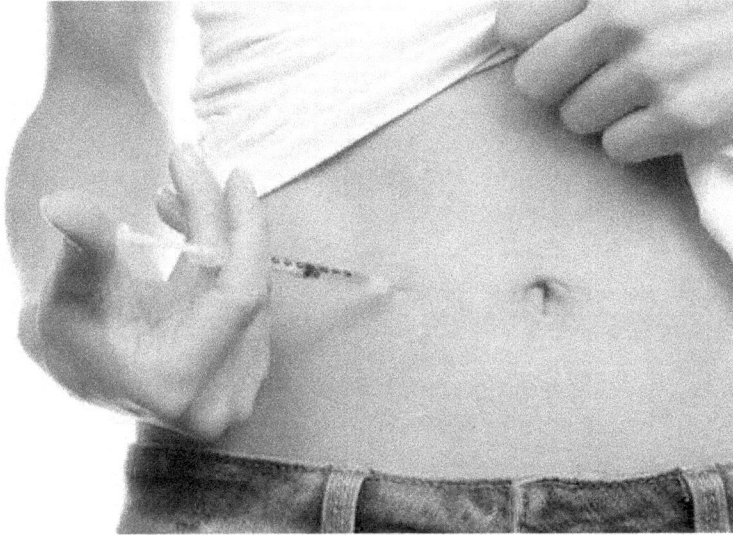

OVERVIEW

Vitamin C serves as a key nutrient necessary for many essential life functions. It provides a crucial role in the treatment of cancer in two ways: by boosting the immune system and by serving as a powerful antioxidant. In 1928, the discovery of Vitamin C was credited to Szent-Gyorgyi ‚Äì a Hungarian biochemist and Nobel Prize winner who ironically enough developed a strong interest in cancer research in his later years. Not long after its discovery, vitamin C began its synthesis and production, thus becoming widely available.

Szent-Gyorgyi perhaps sparked the interest in vitamin C and cancer research, as over the course of time; several case reports and scientific studies were conducted that investigated the effects of vitamin C on cancer. Initially, however, the results of many of these studies were deemed unacceptable, as they were both non-randomized and retrospective.

In the context of cancer, high-dose intravenous vitamin C (> 0.5 g per kg body weight) is claimed to have several effects: a) cytotoxicity for cancer cells, but not for normal tissue, b) improved quality of life for cancer patients, c) protection of normal tissues from toxicity caused by chemotherapy, and d) reinforcement of the action of radiation and some types of chemotherapy.

High-dose vitamin C is essentially non-toxic. Reported side-effects are minor if patients are adequately screened for renal disease and glucose 6-phosphate dehydrogenase deficiency, as well as when doses are slowly increased with careful monitoring of the patient. It should be noted, however, that vitamin C could potentially reduce the effectiveness of conventional cancer treatments.

MECHANISM OF ACTION

At the normal physiological concentrations (e.g., oral doses), vitamin C is an antioxidant that inactivates reactive oxygen species. However, at high, intravenous concentrations, vitamin C is a pro-oxidant, generating hydrogen peroxide that is lethal to cancer cells. In fact, studies indicate that intravenous vitamin C successfully killed cells originating from several cancers. In contrast, oral doses did not. When vitamin C is administered in large, intravenous doses, it undergoes a complex biochemical reaction, with the end result being hydrogen peroxide. In contrast, studies indicate that normal "oral" doses of vitamin C did not result in the formation of hydrogen peroxide. It has been purported that extracellular hydrogen peroxide has the ability to diffuse into cancer cells, mediating toxicity by ATP depletion—of which, results in cancer cell death. In normal cells, hydrogen peroxide is promptly neutralized by various antioxidant enzymes. However, antioxidant enzyme levels are low or imbalanced in most human cancers. As a result, large doses of intravenous vitamin C could potentially serve as a prodrug for the creation of hydrogen peroxide, consequently resulting in the destruction of cancerous cells.

WARNINGS AND SIDE EFFECTS

Essentially, vitamin C is non-toxic. In general, most (if any) adverse events occurring after high-dose intravenous vitamin C were mild and usually preventive by consuming lots of fluids. Nevertheless, doctors advise patients with kidney disease to exercise caution before beginning intravenous vitamin C therapy. The potential exists for negative interactions to occur when vitamin C is added to conventional anti-cancer therapy.

DOSAGE AND ROUTE OF ADMINISTRATION

Vitamin C can be administered via several routes, including orally. In order to be effective for cancer patients, however, it must be administered intravenously. Average dosage amounts for cancer patients range from 10mg-60mg of vitamin C per day—with doses of up to 100mg per day being reported with no adverse side effects.

RESEARCH

Thus far, there have been no randomized controlled clinical trials with published, positive results for high-dose intravenous vitamin C. Nevertheless, a number of Phase I clinical trials confirm the non-toxic nature of the treatment, thereby giving indication and hope to those needing the highest levels of improved quality of life. However, these do not suggest specific anti-cancer properties. Moreover, numerous case reports state that high doses intravenous vitamin C has a positive effect of patient survival time—some even report cancer remission, as well as improved quality of life.

CASE STUDIES

Drisko et al. described two cases of advanced epithelial ovarian cancer. Both patients were first treated with chemotherapy and oral antioxidants, after which 60 g intravenous vitamin C was administered twice weekly for one patient in combination with consolidation paclitaxel chemotherapy. Both patients were disease-free three years after diagnosis. No toxicity was found.[14]

Riordan et al. published case reports for patients with metastasized adenocarcinoma of the kidney, metastasized pancreas cancer, metastasized breast cancer, metastasized stage IV colorectal carcinoma, metastasized carcinoma of the pancreas, and two cases of non-Hodgkin's lymphoma. Vitamin C infusions, as sole treatment or combined with conventional therapy, were generally started at 15g twice weekly and increased to 30 to 100g twice weekly for long periods of time. In all but one case, complete remission was observed. Overall, results indicated lack of toxicity.[15]

MCP

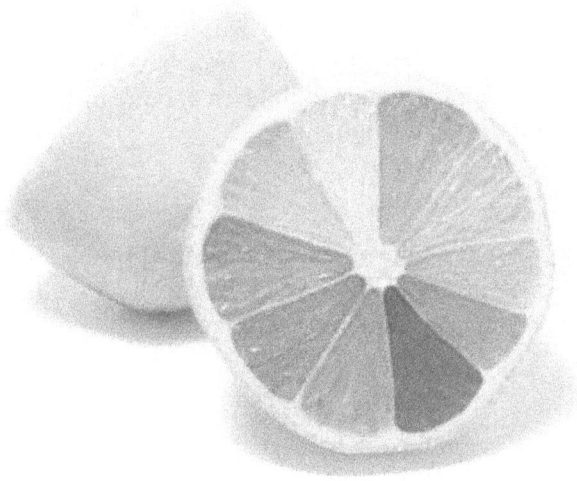

OVERVIEW

Pectin is a type of carbohydrate that is found in the peels of many different plant species—most notably, apples and plums. With modified citrus pectin, however, the pectin undergoes a chemical process that alters its molecular structure, thus reducing its molecules into smaller pieces. The problem with pectin is that in its natural form, it cannot be absorbed by the digestive tract and as a result, cannot easily be absorbed into the bloodstream. Modified citrus pectin, because of its smaller molecule size, can more easily be absorbed by the intestinal tract and the bloodstream.

The popularity of modified citrus pectin came about based on research findings conducted by Dr. Ken Pienta. In his study, Dr. Pienta concluded that modified citrus pectin, when administered orally to rats with prostate cancer, helped stop the metastasis of prostate tumors.

MECHANISM OF ACTION

Proponents claim that modified citrus pectin stop or at least abate the growth of melanoma, a dangerous form of skin cancer, as well as metastatic prostate cancer.

Furthermore, it has been reported that modified citrus pectin strengthens the cancer killing ability of T Cells—cells that also protect against germs.

WARNINGS AND SIDE EFFECTS

There have been no reported cases of any serious adverse reactions resulting from the use of modified citrus pectin. However, people who have allergies or sensitivities to citrus fruits could potentially experience stomach discomfort when taking any form of citrus pectin. According to the FDA, citrus pectin is considered POSSIBLY SAFE for most people, including children and pregnant and breast-feeding women, when used in medicinal amounts.

ADMINISTRATION

Modified citrus pectin is available in both capsule and powder form. The suggested dose for the powder is 5 grams, taken 3 times daily with meals. The suggested regimen for capsules is 800 mg, 3 times daily with meals.

RESEARCH

Several animal studies found that MCP helped reduce the spread of prostate, breast, and skin cancer. Animals with these types of cancer that were fed MCP had a much lower risk of the tumor spreading to the lungs. For example, one study examined the effects of MCP on lung metastases from melanoma cells. Researchers injected mice with melanoma cells. In the mice that were also given MCP, significantly fewer tumors spread to the lungs than in the mice that did not receive the drug. When lung tumors did develop in the mice treated with MCP, the tumors tended to be smaller than those that formed in untreated animals.

These studies appear to show that MCP makes it difficult for cancer cells that break off from the main tumor to join together and grow in other organs. However, in most animal studies, MCP had no effect on the main tumor, suggesting that it may only be useful for preventing or slowing the growth of metastatic tumors in very early stages of development.

Recent laboratory studies of human and animal cells have provided information on how MCP might slow the spread of cancer. MCP appears to attach to galectin-3, a common chemical in many cells. Galectin-3 is present in abnormally high levels in many cancers and plays an important role in the growth, survival, and spread of cancer cells.

Although animal and cell studies are quite encouraging, very little information is available about whether MCP is effective in humans. In one published clinical trial,

10 men with prostate cancer were treated with MCP after standard treatment failed. In 7 of these men, blood tests found prostate-specific antigen (PSA, a marker of prostate cancer growth). Their PSA doubling time (a measure of how fast PSA goes up) improved in comparison with measurements done before taking MCP, indicating that MCP may have a slowing effect on the cancer's growth. This study had no control group (in this case, a group of men who did not take MCP), which limits the strength of its conclusions on MCP's effectiveness. It also did not measure survival or other important endpoints. However, taken with the information gained from animal studies, it suggests that MCP may have a role in reducing the growth and spread of cancer. Randomized controlled trials looking at larger groups of people must be done before any firmer conclusions can be reached.

DEVELOPER

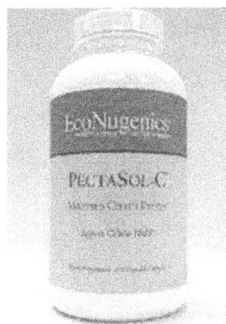

Dr. Kenneth Pienta, Wayne State University Medical School

RETAIL SUPPLIERS

CJ Patton Center
151 Mifflin Road
Miller's Burg, PA 17061
717-362-2067
717-362-3757

Natural Health Consultants
P.O. Box 1091
Vallejo, California 94590
Toll-free: 888 852-4993
Information Hotline: 707 554-1820
Fax: 707 647-3055

Klabin Marketing
2067 Broadway, Suite #700
New York NY 10023
800-933-9440 or 212-877-3632

PRICE

Approximately $90 per month

PAWPAW

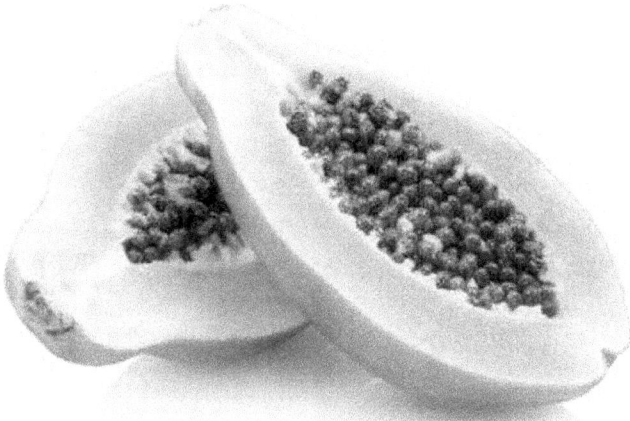

OVERVIEW

The pawpaw is a variety of small fruit trees native to North America, particularly eastern states like Ohio but can also be cultivated as far south as Florida. The fruits of the pawpaw have long been popular as a snack in the eastern states for their soft, creamy flesh that has them dubbed as "Indiana bananas." However, their therapeutic properties have only just been investigated in recent years, as more researchers begin to focus their attention on this humble fruit and its powerful anti-tumor properties.

Much progress in this field was advanced by the research of Jerry McLaughlin, professor of pharmacognosy at Purdue University, who based his life's work on researching extracts from pawpaw. Together with his graduate students, he is responsible for the credibility of pawpaw as a cancer treatment in the scientific community, and the increased effectiveness of pawpaw supplements on the market. He was awarded the Varro Tyler Prize for RESEARCH ON Botanicals by the American Society of Pharmacognosy in 2007.

Pawpaw aids in fighting cancer by altering the production of energy in the body. In every tumor, there are a percentage of cells that become resistant to chemo and multiple drugs. These multiple-drug resistant (MDR) cells continue to multiply and form resistant tumors. Pawpaw works by slowing cell production of energy by blocking adenosine triphosphate (ATP), a molecule that fuels other cell activities. It retards blood circulation around the tumors, and depletes the DNA and RNA components used in cell growth, so that the cancer cells are starved of energy. Pawpaw and its cousin, graviola, are the only two supplements known to be able to kill MDR cells.

Aside from its anti-tumor properties, Pawpaw is known to have anti-viral, anti-fungal and anti-parasitic properties, which is why it is also a component in organic insecticide.

MECHANISM OF ACTION

Pawpaw's effectiveness is attributed to its long carbon chains of atoms, which are called annonaceous acetogenins. Annonaceous acetogenins are what cause the modifications in the body's energy production process described in the OVERVIEW. Acetogenins block the delivery of energy to cancerous cells. This is particularly important as cancer cells divide more rapidly than normal cells by growing more blood vessels to supply nutrients and using ATP to pump drugs out of the cancer cells. Cancer cells hog up to 17 times the energy used by normal cells, simultaneously starving the normal cells while promoting their own duplication.

Acetogenins target these cells with high energy consumption and work to plug the ATP production, causing the cancer cells to lose their energy supply and protection from the drugs. When the ATP levels in cancer cells fall below minimum levels, the cells self-destruct by apoptosis (programmed cell death) or are phagocytized (consumed) by other cells.

WARNINGS AND SIDE EFFECTS

Pawpaw has few side effects but these side effects should be considered when embarking on the treatment. There are also some supplements which counteract its effects and therefore should not be taken at the same time.

1. Nausea and Vomiting
The most commonly reported side effect is nausea. Pawpaw is an emetic, like ipecac, so it may cause patients to throw up, particularly at the beginning. These side effects may lessen with longer use.

2. Risk of Allergy
There is a rare occurrence of allergy to pawpaw, just as natural allergies occur with other forms of food.

3. Not to be taken with CoQ10, thyroid stimulators or antioxidants
Co-enzyme Q10 and certain thyroid medications work to increase energy production which is not desirable as the objective is to starve cancer cells of energy, causing them to go into apoptosis. Antioxidants prevent apoptosis from taking place which is again, not desirable for this treatment, and will reverse the powerful effects of pawpaw.

Pregnant and breastfeeding women are strongly warned not to take pawpaw. As pawpaw works by targeting high-energy cells and starving them of energy, this will be particularly damaging to a fetus which may be seen as a parasite that consumes too much power. For the same reason, healthy patients should not take pawpaw as a preventive supplement as it can disrupt regular cellular functions in the body.

RESEARCH ON PAWPAW

Over 50 unique acetogenins have been discovered in pawpaw extracts using the brine shrimp lethality bioassay, with the potential of more yet to be found. Inclusion of extracts from related species would raise this number to over 150 unique acetogenins. These annonaceous acetogenins derive from long carbon chain fatty acids (C32 or C34). They show powerful effects in stopping complex I (mitochondrial) and anaerobic (cytoplasmic) generation of ATP, as well as DNA and RNA. In addition, a number of acetogenins have been found to operate at high activity at low dosage, which bodes well for its potential as a cancer treatment. Its cytotoxicity has also been noted for potential use in antiviral, antimicrobial, anti-malarial and pesticide products.[16]

NECESSITY OF MEDICAL SUPERVISION

Medical supervision is not required for the self-administration of pawpaw supplements which are naturally derived from edible fruit and pose no danger to health aside from minor side effects. To see best results, people wishing to take Pawpaw should educate themselves on how other supplements can complement or counteract the effects on pawpaw.

RETAIL SUPPLIERS

Healthy Sunshine
http://www.healthy-sunshine.com
506 Ivy Lake Road
Morrison, TN 37357, USA
1-888-523-1727

New Beginnings in Health
http://www.newbeginningsinhealth.com/
8025 Varna Ave
Van Nuys CA 91402, USA
1-877-871-6262

PRICE

A bottle of 180 capsules retails for about $40

EGCG

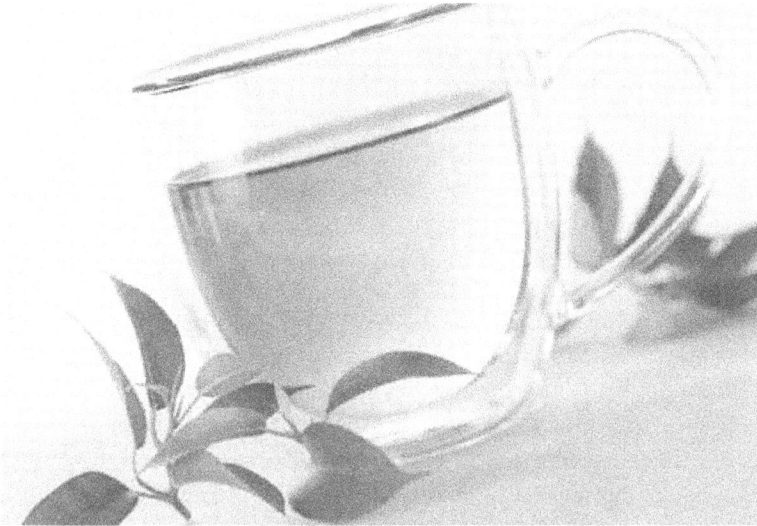

OVERVIEW

Green tea has been known for centuries as a healthy drink, and this knowledge has been backed by scientific research that has found powerful antioxidants in green tea, namely its high concentrations of polyphenols, alkaloids, and other plant-based proteins.

Green tea's health benefits are thought to be attributed to its polyphenols, particularly the catechine epigallocatechin-3-gallate, or EGCG as it is known, which has been shown to have a powerful antioxidant effect as a free radical scavenger. Of all the teas, green tea and white tea contain the most EGCG, as the leaves are unfermented. It is noted that traditionally brewed tea contains the most EGCG, and other types of preparations such as iced teas and bottled teas may not yield the same polyphenol amounts.

Green tea is widely available and is popularly seen as a drink that can prevent cancer. However, substantive evidence behind this claim is still not readily available, as many clinical studies have produced conflicting results, making findings inconclusive. As an anti-cancer agent, researchers have found that EGCG has the potential to induce cell apoptosis, but this has not resulted in the synthesis of a viable anti-cancer drug. Essentially, the field of phytochemicals may not be advanced enough to fully unlock the biological potential of green tea. Therefore, at present, it is best to say that green tea is a safe diet supplement that should be included as part of a supplementary cancer protocol, but should not be relied on as a comprehensive cancer treatment.

MECHANISM OF ACTION

Green tea's anti-cancer properties are attributed to its polyphenols—of which, there are several kinds with high antioxidant activity. Tea polyphenols have a strong protective function. They act as free radical scavengers, protecting cells from having their DNA destroyed by oxidative pollutants and toxins. In addition, they activate enzymes that detoxify the body. Polyphenols have also been proven to inhibit cancerous growth and induce programmed cell death in pre-clinical studies. In addition they may protect against UV damage and boost the body's immunity.

The exact science of how polyphenols work is not known. It is hypothesized that EGCG may interfere with cancer cell-bonding or with communication within cancer cells, thus inhibiting the process of cell multiplication. Through limiting and suppressing growth, EGCG may induce apoptosis in cancer cells. In addition, it is hypothesized that the polyphenols and the other organic agents in green tea may repair free radical damage in cells, restoring them to health, and preventing their mutation into cancer cells.

WARNINGS AND SIDE EFFECTS

The Food and Drug Administration considers green tea to be a safe food product when taken within limits. Safety studies have indicated that 1,200 mg of EGCG over 4 weeks is the upper limit, where side effects like nausea, heart burn, and gastrointestinal issues were reported. A Japanese test found that children were able to consume 576 mg of catechins daily for 24 weeks without side effects.

The caffeine content in green tea may also cause side effects like heart palpitations, insomnia, anxiety, trembling, headaches, nausea, diarrhea, and gastrointestinal upset. The recommended safe level of caffeine consumption is about 300 to 400 mg a day, which is considered moderate by most health authorities.

Although tea is considered a safe product for consumption, pregnant and breastfeeding women should be careful in consuming green tea due to the levels of caffeine present. Because caffeine can pass through breast milk, it may cause sleeplessness in infants. It may also be linked to anemia and a poor ability to metabolize iron.

RESEARCH ON GREEN TEA

Research into green tea is still in its early stages, as is the entire field of phytochemicals. EGCG was isolated as a powerful catechin in 1997 by the Mayo Clinic—of whom, found that it was an active ingredient that could inhibit tumor development and induce apoptosis in human prostate cancer cells.[17] Subsequently, researchers found that EGCG was able to cause apoptosis and DNA breakdown in human epidermis carcinoma cells, prostrate carcinoma cells, and lymphoma cells without causing any damage to normal human epidermal cells, which were the control.[18]

One large study of 472 breast cancer patients found that women who consumed the most green tea experienced the least amount of cancerous growth. In addition, the study found that regular green tea drinkers among the patients enjoyed a lower recurrence rate after achieving remission. However, green tea produced no effects in women who already had advanced stages of breast cancer.[19] These findings should be assessed in comparison with other human clinical trials, which are typically inclusive, possibly due to the large number of human factors involved and the preparation styles of the tea. The general consensus is that more research is required into green tea before scientists can find out how best to use it in a more effective manner to fight cancer.

NECESSITY OF MEDICAL SUPERVISION

No medical supervision is required for the self-administration of green tea, which is a common and safe food. However, people planning to increase their intake of green tea should take note of the warnings about upper limits, as well as the possible health risks of excessive caffeine intake.

RETAILERS

GNC
http://www.gnc.com
Multiple locations
1-877-GNC-4700

The Vitamin Shoppe
http://www.vitaminshoppe.com
Multiple locations
1-866-293-3367

PRICE

Green tea is widely available in supermarkets for a range of prices. Those who wish to avoid caffeine, however, can consider green tea extracts, which are generally caffeine-free and offer a high concentration of catechins and polyphenols. These generally range from $15-20 for 100 capsules.

DHA & EPA

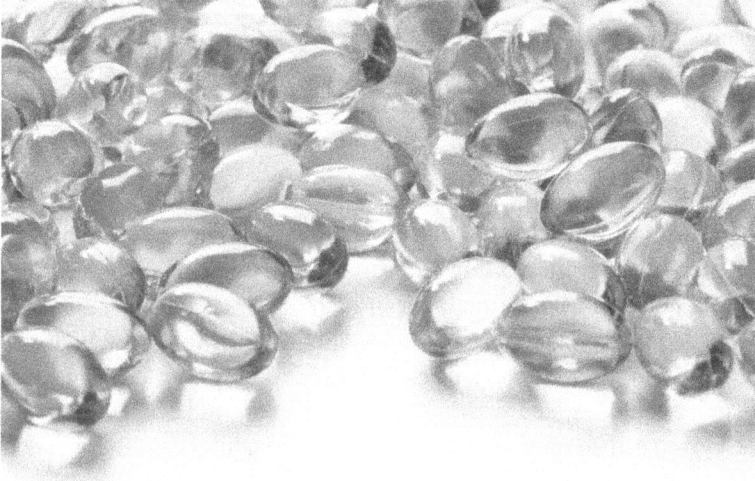

OVERVIEW

DHA and EPA are compounds found in fish oil, particularly, fatty fish. Common types of fatty fish include salmon, tuna, and mackerel. Fish oil is nothing short of a wonder supplement, as it provides superior protection against heart disease, chronic inflammation, depression, and a plethora of other benefits. Accordingly, the consumption of fish and or fish oil, is recommended by many health practitioners, and should be included as part of a well-balanced diet. Fish oil contains what are known as omega-3 fatty acids; specifically, docosahexaenoic acid (DHA) and eicosapentaenoic acid (EPA).

Omega 3 is believed to reduce the risk of cancer.

MECHANISM OF ACTION AND RESEARCH

According to Dr. Barry Sears, author of *The Omega Rx Zone*, fish oil can prove extremely beneficial to cancer patients. Although his claims are backed solely by his personal observations; nevertheless, his voice carries clout, as he is a well-respected member of the medical community. Dr. Sears states that an overabundance of bad eicosanoids (i.e., a derivative of prostaglandins responsible for inflammation and damaging the immune system) weakens the immune system, thus allowing for an increased risk of developing cancer. Consuming high doses of pharmaceutical grade fish oil will increase your levels of eicosapentaenoic acid ‚Äì a chemical necessary to inhibit the formation.

WARNINGS AND SIDE EFFECTS

The FDA states that fish oil is LIKELY SAFE for most people, including pregnant and breast-feeding women, when taken in low doses (3 grams or less per day). This is in contrast, however, to the recommendations set forth below. In addition, fish oil can cause side effects including belching, bad breath, heartburn, nausea, loose stools, rash, and nosebleeds. Taking fish oil supplements with meals or freezing them can often decrease these side effects.

Taking high doses of fish oil is POSSIBLY UNSAFE. Taking more than 3 grams per day might keep blood from clotting and can increase the chance of bleeding. Taking fish oil supplements in larger amounts can increase levels of the "bad" LDL cholesterol in some people. You will need blood tests periodically to ensure LDL cholesterols do not become too high. Some species of fish (e.g., king mackerel and farm-raised salmon) can be contaminated with mercury and other industrial and environmental chemicals. However, fish oil supplements typically do not contain these contaminants.

Potentially harmful contaminants such as dioxins, methylmercury, and polychlorinated biphenyls (PCBs) are found in some species of fish, and may be harmful in pregnant/nursing women. Methylmercury accumulates in fish meat more than in fish oil, and fish oil supplements appear to contain almost no mercury. Therefore, these safety concerns apply to eating fish but likely not to ingesting fish oil supplements. However, unrefined fish oil preparations may contain pesticides.[20]

ADMINISTRATION AND DOSAGE

During Chemotherapy and or Radiation

- 10-15 grams of pharmaceutical-grade fish oil per day

After Treatment

- Reduce intake to 5-10 grams per day of bad eicosanoids. Consequently, your chances of surviving cancer increase greatly.[21]

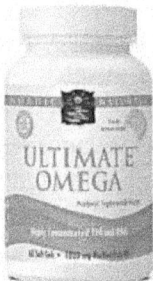

SUPPLIERS

www.nordicnaturals.com

GNC
http://www.gnc.com
Multiple locations
1-877-GNC-4700

SAC & SAMC

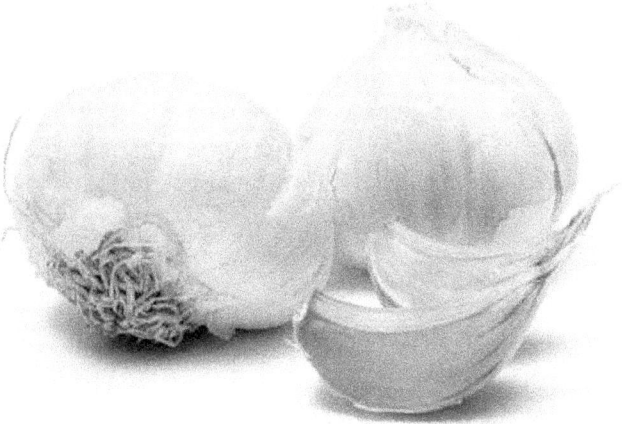

OVERVIEW

Garlic is one of the oldest plants cultivated and consumed by mankind, and it has been renowned for its many medicinal effects for millennia. Unsurprisingly, garlic commands a great deal of interest from the scientific community for its therapeutic potential, particularly for cancer.

Garlic is known in folk wisdom for its anti-tumor properties, and was frequently applied as a poultice on external tumors to shrink them. However, the way the cancer actually worked was a mystery until recently. For example, recent phyto-chemical research has been able to shed light into the therapeutic potential for cancer treatment and identify key compounds that act to suppress cancer growth and cause tumor cell apoptosis.

Innovations in medical techniques are able to take advantage of these compounds by combining them with vaccines or antibodies and infusing them into the tumor tissue. While there are not yet conclusive results for these studies, this is likely to be the future form of garlic-derived treatments. Aside from these treatments, garlic can also be consumed raw or as garlic extracts, and should be considered as dietary supplements to a comprehensive cancer protocol.

MECHANISM OF ACTION

One of the earliest compounds to be identified, allicin, is a major active compound that has anti-bacterial and anti-fungal properties. Recent research has found that allicin is toxic to cancer cells and is also able to induce cell apoptosis and stimulate caspases that target cancer cell production.

In addition to the powerful properties of allicin, researchers have identified another two compounds in aged garlic, S-allylcysteine (SAC) and S-allylmercapto-L-cysteine (SAMC). These exhibit strong free radical properties, while other organosulfur molecules have showed the ability to slow or suppress cancer growth when tested on cancer-bearing animals. These may be promising in terms of cancer prevention.[22]

Lastly, garlic has the ability to stimulate the immune system. Garlic encourages the production of lymphocytes and macrophages, and also triggers the release of interleukins, interferon, and other cells that kill cancer cells. Some early studies also show that garlic can revive or strengthen the healthy immune response, which is important in lowering the risk of cancer.

WARNINGS AND SIDE EFFECTS

Although garlic is a safe and widely-used food that has been used for thousands of years, it should be noted that consumption should be on a moderate basis. Some of the health risks and side effects associated with garlic are:

Too much garlic intake results in strong body odor and bad breath, as well as side effects such as nausea, heartburn, increased insulin production, and diarrhea.

In addition, garlic is a natural blood thinner. Consequently, it should be avoided by pregnant women, those on blood thinning medication, and those awaiting surgery.

Those on prescription drugs should also check if an increased dose of garlic is compatible with their drugs.

Garlic can cause allergies ranging from mild discomfort to anaphylactic shock.

Those taking raw garlic should be careful of taking it on a raw stomach. Also, garlic bulbs can be contaminated by bacteria, which can be dangerous if taken raw.

As mentioned above, while garlic is safe for consumption by pregnant women on a moderate basis, high quantities should be avoided because of its blood thinning qualities.

RESEARCH ON GARLIC

Aged garlic has provoked increased attention from researchers, as the aging process seems to increase the number of antioxidant phytochemicals present that prevent free radical damage. These phytochemicals found in aged garlic extracts include unique organosulfur components and flavonoids. Aged garlic has strong antioxidant abilities and improves the performance of antioxidant enzymes in the cells. It also protects DNA from damage and oxidation.[23]

In addition, research into allicin has produced some recent breakthroughs. Scientists have found an innovative way to deliver allicin directly to tumors, thus ensuring a more powerful and targeted attack on these cancer cells. In a 2003 study, researchers were able to combine the alliinase compound extracted from fresh garlic to an antibody that specifically targeted tumor molecules.. After the antibody was bound to the tumor cell, the scientists were able to trigger the production of allicin, which then killed the tumor cells in vitro, while healthy cells were not affected.[24]

NECESSITY OF MEDICAL SUPERVISION

No medical supervision is necessary for the consumption of garlic, which is a safe and common food. However, those looking to increase their consumption of garlic should be aware of the side effects associated with over consumption. It should also be noted that consumption of raw garlic or extracts should not be relied on as a preventive or cancer-fighting treatment, but used as a supplement.

RETAILERS

GNC
http://www.gnc.com
Multiple locations
1-877-GNC-4700

The Vitamin Shoppe
http://www.vitaminshoppe.com
Multiple locations
1-866-293-3367

PRICE

Raw garlic is inexpensive and widely available. However, those who do not like the unpleasant flavors and odors associated with garlic can consider buying garlic supplements, which cost between $8-15 for 100 capsules

PART TWO:

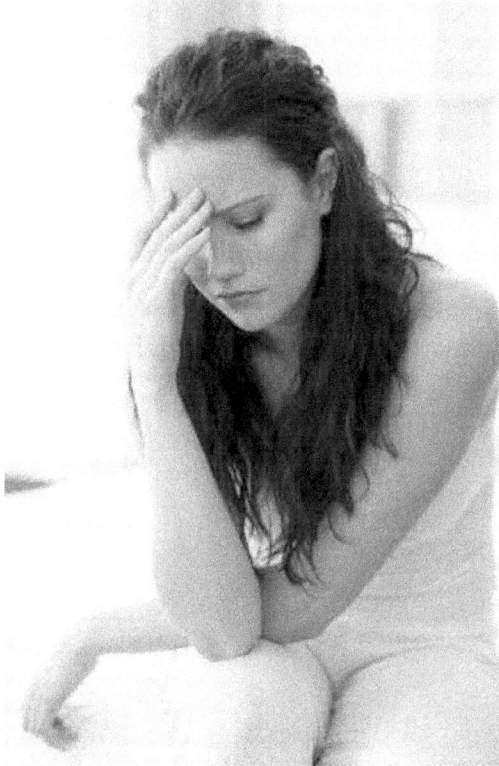

FRAUDULENT TREATMENTS TO AVOID

CELL SPECIFIC CANCER THERAPY (CSCT)

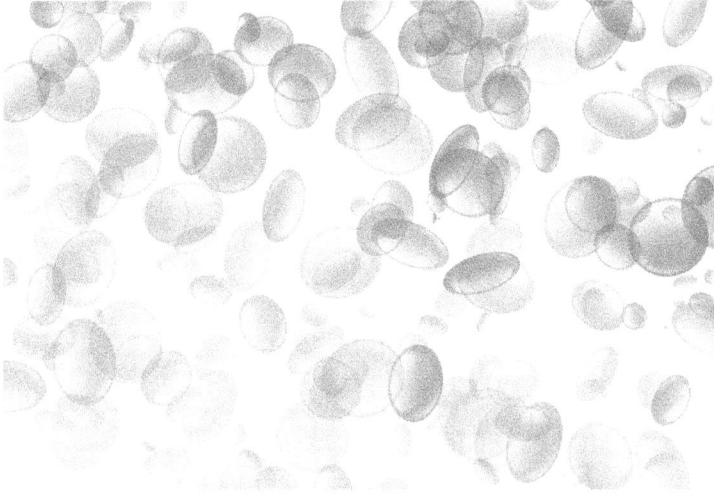

OVERVIEW

The cell-specific-cancer-treatment (CSCT) was potentially the largest fraud operation in the history of alternative cancer treatments. CSCT was administered at a variety of Zoetron therapy centers—which, were eventually shut down by the FTC. The promoters of CSCT therapy—John Armstrong and Michael Reynolds—claimed that a magnetic device could "selectively impact the life cycle of cancerous cells without harming the normal cells in any way." CSCT was originally marketed in London, England, and at CSCT, Inc., in Canada, originally in Kitchener, Ontario. In 1996, the first CSCT facility opened in the Dominican Republic and was later moved to Tijuana, Mexico, in 1998. Cost for the treatment was originally set at $20,000 but was later lowered to $15,000 in 1998. Furthermore, Zoetron therapy centers stated that patients who were unable to afford treatment were eligible for a reduce rate, or potentially, treated free of charge. In 1997, the clinic promised refunds to dissatisfied patients, but later stopped doing this. In 2003, a coordinated effort by government officials in the United States, Canada, and Mexico put the promoters out of business.[25]

MECHANISM OF ACTION

Supporters of CSCT claimed that, in the majority of cases, decrease the amount of damage caused by cancerous cells. Furthermore, they stated that hypothetically, if the total amount of damage caused by cancer cells could be minimized, then that person would have a fighting chance. According to supporters, if a terminal person had a chance to revitalize their immune system, they would detoxify their body as a result, thus increasing the rate of cancer cell death.

In addition, the promoters claimed cancer cells can accumulate iron, and because the CSCT therapy supposedly produced magnetic fields that caused the iron to vibrate and emit heat, the result was the death of cancer cells.[26]

CSCT was purported to be delivered via a ring-like device that was about two feet in diameter and four inches thick. Initially, the patient would lie on a table with his or her body in the ring. During this time, the "therapist" would listen for sounds (produced by the device) that were supposed to indicate the presence of cancer cells. The promoters of CSCT claimed the device could detect differences in the vibrations between cancer cells and healthy cells. Once the cancer cells were detected, the device would kill the cancer cells by disrupting their frequency—of which, would cause them to rupture and die.[27]

WARNINGS AND SIDE EFFECTS

Physical side effects were essentially non-existent during CSCT therapy. However, the financial strain caused by this swindle operation, coupled with the amount of mental anguish endured by the unfortunate patients, probably resulted in long-term emotional and financial consequences.

RESEARCH

Promoters of CSCT published many case histories, as well as two summary reports, in which explanations for the efficacy of CSCT treatment are purported to be outlined. However, the reports failed to utilize appropriate scientific methods for evaluating the results of cancer treatment, and as a result, should be disdained as futile. Similarly, no conclusion could be obtained from the individual case reports, as they outlined insufficient data that later proved to be worthless, as well.

For example, one such summary report was comprised of 50 patients from the Netherlands—of whom, were treated between 1996 and 1999. The data were reviewed in a table that listed treatment results as: 1.favorable, 2. unfavorable, 3. indefinite, or 4. other. The result was 23 cases, 7 cases, 16 cases, and 4 cases, respectively. Moreover, concluding evidence suggested that the report defined these terms. However, it delivered no raw data to permit the reader to determine: 1. in what way the criteria were applied, 2. by what means the patient follow-up status was obtained, 3.which patients had formerly undergone conventional therapy, and 4. which patients were alive at the time of compilation. In addition, although the table included information about the stage (seriousness) of each cancer, it did not indicate as to when the staging was complete. The final, official quote from the report follows:

"The evidence presented here is not yet conclusive of the efficacy of the CSCT/ Zoetron therapy." It would be more accurate to state that the data have no significance whatsoever.[28]

GOVERNMENT ACTION

In 2003, the Federal Trade Commission gained a provisional restraining order that banned John Leslie Armstrong and Michael John Reynolds—the founders of the operation—from enduring asinine claims as to the effectiveness of CSCT therapy. Furthermore, when they went to trial, the judge froze their resources and instructed them to close their website. A copy of the official complaint that was subpoenaed into court is listed below:

During the patient's stay at the clinic, staffers claim to assess the patient's condition by analyzing tumor size, blood chemistry, and tumor markers. As time goes by, the clinic may tell a patient that his or her tumor has reduced in size or that their tumor marker tests are decreasing. If a consumer expresses some doubt, possibly because the consumer's observation of the tumor indicates that there is no change, the clinic will assure . . . that the cancerous cells are in fact dead and explain . . . that the body simply takes time to eliminate the dead cancerous cells.[29]

The decision to shut down the CSCT operation was directed by police and federal agencies in Canada and Mexico. Ultimately, it was Mexico's Ministry of Health that shut down the CSCT operation, after it was found that the clinic offered swindle treatments to poor, unsuspecting people. According to Canadian, US, and Mexican government officials, it is believed that approximately 850 people had received CSCT treatment across a span of 5 years. Later, in 1994, the three nations launched a health fraud work group in order to enhance their ability to fight fraud treatment companies that operate within one country, targeting unsuspecting patients who live in another.

Ultimately, in 2004, CSCT, Inc. signed a consent agreement that banned them from advertising CSCT therapy. In addition, the settlement contained a judgment worth $7.6 million—of which, was suspended, as the defendants stated that they couldn't pay it. Afterwards, the FTC complied, realizing they were in no way capable of paying the fine. Finally, the settlement prohibited John Leslie Armstrong and Michael John Reynolds from selling information concerning anybody whose data was obtained in association with the advertising or distribution of their services.[30]

ESSIAC TEA

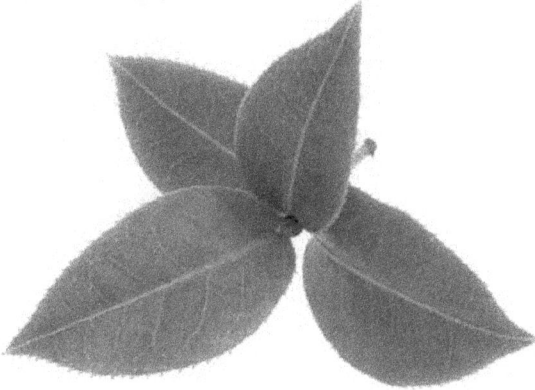

OVERVIEW

Originally consisting of four herbs—burdock root, slippery elm inner bark, sheep sorrel, and Indian rhubarb root—Essiac is mixture of herbs that are combined to make a tea. Four additional herbs—watercress, blessed thistle, red clover, and kelp—were added to later recipes to make a product known as Flor Essence.

In 1922, a Canadian nurse named Rene Caisse learned about the Essiac treatment from one of her patients. The patient claimed that an Indian herbal tea —developed by an Ojibwa medicine man—had freed her from breast cancer. In 1924, Caisse opened a clinic and began to offer cancer patients her newfound herbal tonic—of which, she named Essiac. Essiac is her last name spelled backward. Caisse went on to treat thousands of patients using her innovative herbal mixture as both a tea and an injection. However, in 1938 Canadian medical authorities investigated the clinic and concluded that the Essiac formula offered little evidence towards treating cancer. In 1977, Caisse gave her formula to a manufacturer in Toronto with the intent of selling it for a reasonable price. She died a year later.

MECHANISM OF ACTION

Perhaps the most asinine aspect of treatment with Essiac tea is that Ms. Caisse "theorized" that an herb in Essiac reduced tumor growth and the other herbs served as blood cleansers, disposing of tissue by products, as well as infections related to cancer. In addition, Ms. Caisse hypothesized that Essiac enhanced the body's innate defense mechanisms, thus enabling normal cells to destroy cancerous cells.

WARNINGS AND SIDE EFFECTS

According to one manufacturer of Essiac tea, users may experience increased bowel movements, frequent urination, swollen glands, skin blemishes, flu-like symptoms, or slight headaches. Serious side effects, however, are uncommon. Rarely, serious allergic reactions have been reported. In addition, the potential interactions between Essiac and other drugs and herbs should be considered.

ADMINISTRATION

The typical dosage instructions are based on a "unit" of Essiac tea. For example, a unit of Essiac power makes approximately 72 oz. of Essiac tea. Normal doses vary from 4 to 9 oz., so one unit produces anywhere from 8 to 16 days of tea. The recommended minimum duration of treatment for cancer is 12 weeks.

Women who are pregnant or nursing are advised not to consume Essiac tea, as the potential adverse effects towards the fetus have not been well established by the FDA. In addition, it is advised that if you are taking prescription medications, you should consult with your physician prior to beginning treatment with Essiac tea.

RESEARCH

Research of the anti-cancer effects of Essiac was conducted in 1959 and again in the 1970's. The Memorial Sloan-Kettering Cancer Center conducted animal testing of Essiac; however, no anti-cancer effects were documented. Furthermore, in 1983, Canadian Federal Health officials requested that Essiac be tested by the U.S. National Cancer Institute—of which, found no evidence of anti-cancer activity in animal studies. Moreover, Canadian Federal Health officials—upon reviewing 86 case studies—concluded that the Essiac treatment showed no evidence of abating the progression of cancer. They did note, however, that Essiac users experienced very few, if any, serious side effects, and that the only potential benefit was that of a placebo effect.

Essiac's purported effect on cancer has been reviewed by several No major medical or scientific organizations—including the U.S. Food and Drug Administration, the National Cancer Institute, and the American Cancer Society—support the anti-cancer claims made by Essiac. All have found no evidence that Essiac has any plausible effect (other than perhaps a placebo effect) against cancer. Despite the enormous amount of unproven claims, Essiac still remains a popular anti-cancer treatment. As a result, you should be mindful of the literature when deciding on an alternative cancer treatment.

RETAILERS

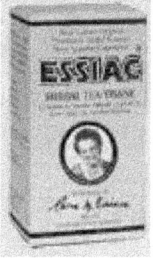

Kevin T. Maloney, INC.
c/o Essiac Canada International
P.O. Box 365
Lake Worth, FL 33460

PRICE

Between $50 and $95 for a 1 month supply.

PROTOCEL/CANTRON

OVERVIEW

The liquid formula known as Protocel, Cantron, Entelev, Cancell or Sheridan's Formula has had a controversial history due to legal battles between rivaling manufacturers over the composition of their products and the right to market and sell them. Today, the updated version of this formula is mainly manufactured and marketed as Protocel or Cantron in the US, and Entelev in Australia.

Protocel/Cantron was formulated in the 1930s by biochemist James V. Sheridan, a biochemist who dispensed it to cancer sufferers free of charge, before deciding to market it as Entelev. The exact composition of the formula is not known as the manufacturers each have their own proprietary blend consisting of different ratios. It is known to consist of electrolytes, vitamins and minerals. The FDA has publicly listed its chemical ingredients to be inositol, nitric acid, sodium sulphite, potassium hydroxide, sulphuric acid and catechol.

Similar to the concept of Pawpaw, Protocel/Cantron works by altering biological processes in the body to deprive cancer cells of energy, causing them to break down as part of apoptosis (programmed cell death) or being eliminated by the body as foreign substances. Sheridan felt that changing the reactions of ion energies would cause the development of cancer cells to reverse, and developed his formula.

Unlike Pawpaw however, the scientific process of the treatment is not clearly known due to the lack of clinical trials and published scientific results. There is however anecdotal reports that Protocel and Cantron have the ability to treat cancer, AIDS, viruses, herpes and unclog arteries. There has also been no severe side effects reported, making it a generally safe and non-toxic choice of treatment.

MECHANISM OF ACTION

Like pawpaw and graviola, Protocel/Cantron works by blocking the production of ATP, causing the cells to receive less energy. What is different about the process, however, is that the chemical composition of the formula causes a reduction of the electrical voltage in the blood from the normal levels of 70 to 110 mv to close to 50 mv. At this level, normal cells still operate as normal. However, energy hogs like cancer cells and viral cells do not get enough energy and begin to starve. When their energy levels fall below critical rates, they will go into apoptosis or be broken down by other cells.

Advocates of this treatment caution that this particular chemical reaction is very sensitive and any disruption caused by the use of other clashing treatments will interfere with its intended manipulation of electrical ions. Therefore, this product comes with strict guidelines on what can be consumed with it that has to be adhered to.

WARNINGS AND SIDE EFFECTS

As earlier noted, there are few reports of side effects to this product. Manufacturers note that there may be tiredness, and there have been a few reports of nausea.

The main warning about this product is essentially its restrictiveness in terms of dietary supplements. Supplements that are not allowed include Vitamin C, Vitamin E, Selenium, CoQ10, Omega-3 Fatty Acids, Essiac Tea, Burdock Root and many others. They are believed to interfere with the electrical processes and energy production in the cells, which will prevent Protocel/Cantron from meeting its specified objective.

This can be a source of inconvenience to those who require such supplements for their nutrition, or who hope to use multiple treatment approaches concurrently.

Buyers should also note that the sale of this product is also controlled by the FDA which considers the product to be unproven. The sale of this product across states is restricted.

While there is not clinical data on this, it is not recommended for pregnant and breastfeeding women to take Protocel or Cantron on the principle that the formula aims to starve cells of energy, which is not suitable for fetal development.

RESEARCH ON PROTOCEL/CANTRON

Lab tests commissioned by the manufacturers of Cantron found Cantron to be a powerful antioxidant, able to scavenge multiple varieties of free radicals that caused disease, as compared to conventional antioxidants like Vitamin C that only worked on one variety. It was noted to be more effective than vitamin E, vitamin C, caffeic acid, green tea and Peroxynitrite.[31]

However, it should be noted that these results were not published in a scientific journal and verified by other independent researchers.

NECESSITY OF MEDICAL SUPERVISION

As Protocel and Cantron are non-toxic and relatively free of side effects, no medical supervision is needed for self-administration.

RETAILERS

WebND
http://www.webnd.com/index.php
3100 Grandview Drive,
Simpsonville, SC 29681, USA
1-888-581-4422

Medical Research Products
www.cantron.com
10873 NW 52nd St
Unit Bay 7 & 8
Sunrise, FL 33351-8000 USA
Toll-free: 1-800-443-3030
Local: 1-954-641-0981

PRICE

The formula is available only in liquid form and costs about $180 for a 274 ml bottle (4 month supply).

GERMANIUM-132

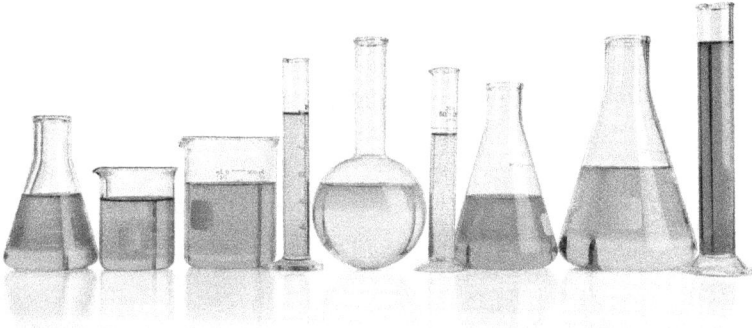

OVERVIEW

Germanium-132 is a mineral that is a powerful antioxidant, able to boost the body's immunity and cancer-fighting ability by encouraging the creation of natural white blood and T-suppressor cells and acting as a catalyst for increased oxygen conversion for the body. As an inorganic element, Germanium is toxic and not suitable for consumption. It is however widely used in semi-conductors and electronic components. However, organic Germanium is also found in a variety of foods and has no toxicity.

An organic Germanium product, Germanium-132 (bis-carboxyethyl germanium sesquioxid), was subsequently created by Japanese chemist Dr.Kazuhiko Asai. This product was found to be similar to the organic Germanium found in wonder foods like ginseng, garlic and aloe.

Pure organic Germanium-132 is safe but the problem regarding Germanium products on the market is that many are tainted by inorganic Germanium, which is toxic. Due to the reported cases of kidney damage from people who took contaminated Germanium-based products, the Food and Drug Administration decided to ban imports of overseas Germanium supplements. USA-made Germanium-132 supplements of high-purity however are available and legal to buy. Consumers are advised to exercise caution when purchasing Germanium products.

MECHANISM OF ACTION

Organic Germanium-132 helps in cancer-fighting in two main immunity-boosting ways. Firstly, Germanium-132 stimulates the growth of cells that target and kill cancer cells, such as Interferon, Macrophages and NK-Lymphocytes, as well as T-suppressor cells.

The other way that Germanium aids in killing cancer cells is by increasing the supply and absorption of oxygen in the body. This is important because studies have found that cancer cells have difficulty metabolizing oxygen. Thus being able to increase the oxygen absorption in cells can possibly retard the growth of cancer cells. Organic germanium also gives up its electrons easily to surrounding molecules. This allows it to operate as a free radical scavengerwhich can neutralize free radicals in the body.

WARNINGS AND SIDE EFFECTS

The Food and Drug Administration considers the consumption of Germanium supplements a potential health hazard due to possible contamination byinorganic Germanium, and has banned the import of Germanium-containing products used for consumption. However, it should be noted that Germanium found naturally in food has no toxic effects. The following risks and warnings are summarized:

1. Risk of Kidney Damage and Toxic Effects
Inorganic Germanium is toxic and should not be consumed. The accumulation of toxins will cause kidney damage (nephrotoxicity), and in extreme cases, death. While organic Germanium is considered safe, buyers must be bewareof products, particularly imports, which may be contaminated.

2. Other Side Effects
Some minor side effects have been reported. One complaint by some patients in a medical study was for softened stools, although this effect ceased after treatment was stopped. Other anecdotal reports noted that long-term usage can cause disruption in sleep patterns or mental performance.

CONSUMPTION IN POWDER FORM

Some advocates of Germanium-132 recommend taking it in powder form as a safer and more reliable way to ensure the lack of side effects. These reasons are:

Increased purity in the powder form, as compared to capsules and tablets that are mixed with other ingredients.

- Powder can be tested for purity by complete dissolution in warm water. The solution should be colorless with no residue or suspension. In comparison, there is no way to test the purity of tablets.

- Powder is consumed by mixing with water and is easily digested. In comparison, the hard coatings on tablets take a long time to be broken down by the digestive system.

RESEARCH ON GERMANIUM-132

Predominantly, researchers noted that Germanium-132 was easily absorbed and discharged by the body without evidence of toxic poisoning. In addition, it has been observed to be an effective free radical scavenger. Organic Germanium consists of 32 electrons, with 4 in an outer ring. These electrons easily bond with other molecules, which have been suggested to be a factor in its antioxidant properties. One medical trial found that the combined intake of Germanium-132 and Selenium reduced the production of hydroxyl free radical.[32]

In addition, other research has found some evidence of tumor-fighting activity. Researchers noted that Germanium-132 can intercalate with DNA to produce an "unexpected methyl substitution effect of the novel derivatives on DNA sequence selectivity and cytotoxicity."[33]

NECESSITY OF MEDICAL SUPERVISION

No medical supervision is required for the consumption of Germanium although patients should take pains to ensure that they obtain a pure organic product from a reputable source. Patients should also do necessary research into a complementary diet and supplements for best results.

There has been little research conducted on pregnant or breast-feeding cases. However, given the risks associated with the purity of organic Germanium products, pregnant or breast-feeding women should not take Germanium.

RETAIL SUPPLIERS

Germanium Inc.
http://www.egermanium.com
176 Jackson Ave.
Syosset, NY 11791, USA

Nutricology
http://www.nutricology.com/

2300 North Loop Road
Alameda, CA 94502, USA
1-800-545-9960

iHerb.com
http://www.iherb.com/
17825 Indian Street
Moreno Valley, CA 92551, USA
1-951-616-3600

PRICE

Ranging from $40 for a bottle of 100 tablets to $2,499 for a 1,000 gram bottle of organic powder.

THE HOXSEY TREATMENT

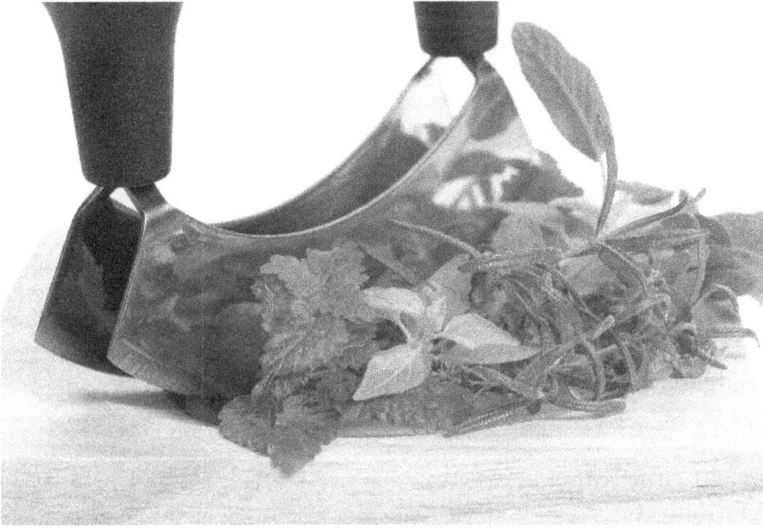

OVERVIEW

The Hoxsey Treatment is a controversial herbal folk remedy that despite widespread denouncement by the scientific community and the Food and Drug Administration, continues to be popular as an alternative cancer treatment. Primarily the treatment consists of two herbal mixtures, a liquid tonic to be consumed, and a salve that should be rubbed onto the skin closest to the tumor. It was popularized by Harry M. Hoxsey, who claimed that his grandfather created the formula in 1840 after observing a farm horse that cured itself from cancer by consuming a number of herbs and grass.

Hoxsey was convicted multiple times for operating a clinic without a medical license and the Food and Drug Administration finally issued a total ban on the treatment in 1960. While the general scientific consensus is that the Hoxsey Treatment is not effective in curing cancer, modern research has revealed that the herbs used may contain natural anti-tumor plant agents like nitrilosides that may work in animals, although in their current form they have little or no effect in humans.

MECHANISM OF ACTION

The liquid tonic in the Hoxsey Treatment consists of red clover, licorice, burdock root, poke root, prickly ash bark, barberry root, cascara, stillingia root, buckthorn bark and potassium iodide. The salve is made from a paste of bloodroot, antimony, arsenic, zinc, sulphur and talc. The actual list of ingredients and ratio may vary from patient to patient and as used by practitioners.

According to the manufacturer, these formulas work by balancing internal body fluids that have stopped self-regulating. However, the actual scientific process is not explained and has not been proven by any medical studies.

Aside from these two mixtures, patients undergoing treatment are usually prescribed nutritional supplements, laxatives, and douches.

CONTROVERSIAL HISTORY

The founder of the Hoxsey Treatment, Harry Hoxsey was a controversial figure who persisted in running clinics in multiple states and prescribing his cure, leading to three convictions. Eventually, after the treatment was banned, he opened his medical center in Mexico. Hoxsey was diagnosed with prostate cancer in 1967. Unsuccessful in curing himself with his own treatment, he had to undergo conventional therapy before passing away seven years later in 1974.

The Food and Drug Administration has banned the Hoxsey Treatment as a "worthless and discredited treatment" since 1960. The treatment is only now available at the Bio-Medical Centre in Tijuana, Mexico, which is run by staff of the late Harry Hoxsey. It should be noted that this center is monitored by Mexican health authorities and has been subjected to mandatory closure in the past for about a month and a half in 2000.

SIDE EFFECTS

The ingredients used in the Hoxsey Treatment have been associated with the following side effects:

- Burns and disfigurement caused by the caustic nature of the salve and tonic
- Nausea, trembling, diarrhea and cramps from laxative effects of buckthorn and cascar
- Aches, palpitations and fatigue from licorice
- Gland inflammations, acne, infections from overdosing on iodine

While Red Clover has anti-carcinogenic properties, it is not suitable for people who take anti-coagulants and for women with estrogen-responsive tumors.

RESEARCH ON THE HOXSEY TREATMENT

Multiple studies carried out by scientific institutions such as, the Food and Drug Administration, MD Anderson Cancer Center and the Memorial Sloan-Kettering

Cancer Centre have found no proof of the Hoxsey Treatment's effectiveness in fighting cancer. In additional, a damning review by the FDA found that many of the 400 patients on the list submitted by Harry Hoxsey did not have cancer at all, while none of those with active cancer were actually cured.

A more recent attempt to track the survival rates of patients who had undergone treatment at the Bio-Medical Center found poor record-keeping. Only 43.6% had actually been given biopsies to test for tumors, follow-up data for many patients were missing and the majority of patients had already received conventional cancer treatments, leading the team to state that any comparative studies were impossible.

It should be noted that modern research does indicate that many of the herbs used in Hoxsey's remedy do have anti-tumor qualities that deserve furtherresearch. One example is a form of the Red Clover that showed some cancer suppression in cell cultures. These findings indicate that there may be some merit in further investigation plants used in folk remedies. However, this does not change the fact that these herbs in their current form are most likely ineffective when used in cases of cancer.

NECESSITY OF MEDICAL SUPERVISION

While the Hoxsey Treatment is banned in the USA, there are alternative practitioners that offer variations of the treatment to be carried out at home. However, the scientific legitimacy is dubious at best and people considering this treatment should proceed with extreme caution.

Pregnant and breastfeeding women are strongly advised not to use the treatment either as pokeweed has been known to cause toxic and fatal reactions in children.

PRACTITIONER

Bio-Medical Center
615 General Ferreira, Colonia Juarez
Tijuana, B.C., Mexico
011-52-664-684-90-11
Mailing Address:
PO Box 433654
San Isidro, CA 92143-3654

PRICE

The cost of treatment ranges between $3,900 and $5,100. Dietary supplements, lab tests and further exams cost extra.

BIBLIOGRAPHY

GENETICALLY ENGINEERED T CELLS

[1]Fred Hutchinson Cancer Research Center: http://www.fhcrc.org/about/ne/news/2008/06/18/T_cells.html

[2]Porter,DL; Levine, BL, et al. "Chimeric Antigen Receptor–Modified T Cells in Chronic Lymphoid Leukemia" The New England Journal of Medicine, August 10, 2011 (10.1056/NEJMoa1103849)

UKRAIN

[3]Ernst, K; Schmidt, E. "Ukrain – a new cancer cure? A systematic review of randomised clinical trials." BMC Cancer. 2005; 5: 69. DOI: 10.1186/1471-2407-5-69

[4]Lanvers-Kaminsky, C; Nolting, D-M, et al. "In-vitro toxicity of Ukrain against human Ewing tumor cell lines ." Anti-Cancer Drugs: October 2006 - Volume 17 - Issue 9 - pp 1025-1030. DOI: 10.1097/01.

[5]Gagliano, N; Moscheni, C, et al. " Effect of Ukrain on matrix metalloproteinase-2 and Secreted Protein Acidic and Rich in Cysteine (SPARC) expression in human glioblastoma cells" Anti-Cancer Drugs: February 2006 - Volume 17 - Issue 2 - pp 189-194

GRAVIOLA

[6]Dai, Y & Hogan, S, et al. "Nutrition and Cancer elective Growth Inhibition of Human Breast Cancer Cells by Graviola Fruit Extract In Vitro and In Vivo Involving Down-regulation of EGFR Expression." Nutrition and Cancer, Volume 63, Issue 5, 2011 pages 795-801. DOI: 10.1080/01635581.2011.563027

[7]Hattori, Masao & Li, CJ et al. "Annonaceous acetogenins from the Leaves of *Annona montana*" Bioorganic & Medicinal Chemistry, Volume 10, Issue 3, March 2002, Pages 561-565

MEDICAL OZONE

[8]Sweet, F; Kao, MS et al. "Ozone selectively inhibits growth of human cancer cells." Science, 209 *4459):921-3. DOI: 10.1126/science.7403859

[9]Bocci, B; Luzzi, E, et al. " Studies on the biological effects of ozone: 5. Evaluation of immunological parameters and tolerability in normal volunteers receiving ambulatory autohaemotherapy" Biotherapy , Volume 7, Number 2, 83-90. DOI: 10.1007/BF01877731

[10]Clavo, B; Pérez, JL, et al. "Ozone Therapy for Tumor Oxygenation: A Pilot Study". Evidence-based Complementary and Alternative Medicine 2004;1(1)93-98, Oxford University Press

HYPERTHERMIA (ONCOTHERMIA)

[11]Wust, P; Hildebrandt, B, et al. "Hyperthermia in combined treatment of cancer." The Lancet Oncology, Volume 3, Issue 8, August 2002. Pages 487-497. DOI: 10.1016/S1470-2045(02)00818-5

[12]Tseng, HY; Lee, GB, et al. "Localised heating of tumours utilising injectable magnetic nanoparticles for hyperthermia cancer therapy." Nanobiotechnology, IET, Vol3, Issue 2, 2008 Pages 46-54. DOI: 10.1049/iet-nbt.2008.0013

[13]Westermann, M; Grosen, EA, et al. "A pilot study of whole body hyperthermia and carboplatin in platinum-resistant ovarian cancer" European Journal of Cancer, Volume 37, Issue 9, 2001, Pages 1111-1117. DOI: 10.1016/S0959-8049(01)00074-0

[14]Drisko JA, Chapman J, Hunter VJ. The use of antioxidants with first-line chemotherapy in two cases of ovarian cancer. J. Am. Coll. Nutr. 2003 April;22(2):118-123.

[15]Riordan HD, Casciari JJ, González MJ, Riordan NH, Miranda-Massari JR, Taylor P, Jackson JA. A pilot clinical study of continuous intravenous ascorbate in terminal cancer patients. P R Health Sci. J. 2005;24(4):269-76.

PAW-PAW

[16]McLaughlin, JL. "Paw Paw and Cancer: Annonaceous Acetogenins from Discovery to Commercial Products", Journal of Natural Products, 2008, ACS Publications. Online source: http://pubs.acs.org/doi/abs/10.1021/np800191t

EGCG

[17]Adrian G. Paschkaa, Rachel Butler and Young, CYF. "Induction of apoptosis in prostate cancer cell lines by the green tea component, (–)-epigallocatechin-3-gallate." Cancer Letters Volume 130, Issues 1-2, 14 August 1998, Pages 1-7

[18]Ahmad, N; Feyes, DK, et al. "Green Tea Constituent Epigallocatechin-3-Gallate and Induction of Apoptosis and Cell Cycle Arrest in Human Carcinoma Cells" *JNCI J Natl Cancer Inst* (1997) 89 (24): 1881-1886. DOI: 10.1093/jnci/89.24.1881

[19]National Cancer Institute factsheet: http://www.cancer.gov/cancertopics/factsheet/prevention/tea

[20]http://www.mayoclinic.com/health/fish-oil/NS_patient-fishoil/DSECTION=safety

[21]*The Omega Rx Zone.* Dr. Barry Sears, M.D. 2002. Harper Collins, New York, NY.

SAC & SAMC

[22]Thomson M.; Ali M.Garlic [Allium sativum]: A Review of its Potential Use as an Anti-Cancer Agent Current Cancer Drug Targets, Volume 3, Number 1, February 2003 , pp. 67-81(15) (*Journal of Nutrition.* 2001;131:1067S-1070S.)

[23]Borek, Carmia. "Antioxidant Health Effects of Aged Garlic Extract" Journal of Nutrition. 2001;131:1010S-1015S.)

[24]Miron, T; Mironchik, M, et al. "Inhibition of tumor growth by a novel approach: In situ allicin generation using targeted alliinase delivery" *Molecular Cancer Therapy* December 2003 2; 1295

[25]Leviton R. Killing cancer cells with magnetic energy. Alternative Medicine Digest, Issue #20, 1996.

[26]Leviton R. Killing cancer cells with magnetic energy. Alternative Medicine Digest, Issue #20, 1996.

[27]Leviton R. Killing cancer cells with magnetic energy. Alternative Medicine Digest, Issue #20, 1996.

[28]Complaint for permanent injunction and other equitable relief. Federal Trade Commission v CSCT, Inc., et al. U.S. District Court for the Northern District of Illinois, Eastern Diviision, Civil No. 03000880, filed Feb 6, 2003.

[29]FTC, Canada, and Mexico officials crack down on foreign companies that offer bogus cancer treatment. FTC news release, Feb 20, 2003.

[30]FTC, Canada, and Mexico officials crack down on foreign companies that offer bogus cancer treatment. FTC news release, Feb 20, 2003.

[31]Hetrick, Daniel, PhD, A study and comprehensive discussion of the antioxidant power of Cantron® including all versions and variations such as Entelev, Cancell and Protocel, 2003, Catron Source: http://www.cantron.com/html/cantron_antioxi_intro.html

GERMANIUM-132

[32]Shangguan, G., Xing, F., Qu, X., Mao, J., Zhao, D., Zhao, X. and J. Ren. "DNA binding specificity and cytotoxicity of novel antitumor agent Ge132 derivatives." Bioorganic & medicinal chemistry letters. Vol. 15, Issue 12. (2962-5). 2005 Jun 15. Available: http://www.ncbi.nlm.nih.gov/entrez/query.fcgi?CMD=search&DB=pubmed PMID: 15914003 [PubMed - indexed for MEDLINE]

[33]Kaplan, B. J., Parish, W. W., Andrus, G. M., Simpson, J. S. and C. J. Field. "Germane facts about germanium sesquioxide: I. Chemistry and anticancer properties." Journal of alternative and complementary medicine. Vol. 10, Issue 2. Apr 2004. (337-44). Available: http://www.ncbi.nlm.nih.gov/entrez/query.fcgi?CMD=search&DB=pubmed PMID: 15165414 [PubMed - indexed for MEDLINE]

www.ingramcontent.com/pod-product-compliance
Lightning Source LLC
Chambersburg PA
CBHW070409200326
41518CB00011B/2132